DREAD

DREAD

HOW FEAR AND FANTASY
HAVE FUELED EPIDEMICS FROM THE
BLACK DEATH TO AVIAN FLU

PHILIP ALCABES

PublicAffairs
New York

Published in the United States by PublicAffairs™,
a member of the Perseus Books Group.

The lines from Thucydides' *Histories*, Book 2, originally translated by P. J. Rhodes, as modified by G. E. R. Lloyd in *The Grip of Disease: Studies in the Greek Imagination* (Oxford, 2003), appear here with permission of Oxford University Press and Aris & Phillips Publications.

Portions of chapter 6 originally appeared in different form in *The American Scholar* (2006).

PublicAffairs books are available at special discounts for bulk purchases in the U.S. by corporations, institutions, and other organizations. For more information, please contact the Special Markets Department at the Perseus Books Group, 2300 Chestnut Street, Suite 200, Philadelphia, PA 19103, call (800) 810-4145, ext. 5000, or e-mail special .markets@perseusbooks.com.

Designed by Trish Wilkinson
Text set in 11.5 point Goudy

Library of Congress Cataloging-in-Publication Data

Alcabes, Philip.
    Dread : how fear and fantasy have fueled epidemics from the black death to avian flu / Philip Alcabes. — 1st ed.
        p. ; cm.
    Includes bibliographical references and index.
    ISBN 978-1-58648-618-1 (alk. paper)
    1. Epidemics—History. 2. Communicable diseases—History. 3. Epidemics—Psychological aspects. 4. Epidemics—Social aspects. 5. Nosophobia. I. Title.
    [DNLM: 1. Disease Outbreaks—history. 2. Fear—psychology. 3. Anxiety—psychology. 4. Communicable Disease Control. 5. Communicable Diseases—history. 6. Health Behavior. WA 11.1 A346d 2009]
    RA649.A43 2009
    614.4—dc22   2009000248

2

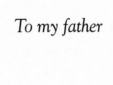

To my father

CONTENTS

THE ORIGINS OF DREAD

Death in it self is nothing; but we fear
To be we know not what, we know not where.
—John Dryden, Aureng-Zebe (1675)

Epidemics fascinate us. Look at all the ways we offer accounts of epidemics, and how often. There are thousands of books in print about epidemics. There are histories of epidemics past, like the Black Death of the 1340s, the yellow fever outbreaks of 1793, cholera in the mid-1800s, the Spanish Flu pandemic of 1918, and polio in the mid-twentieth century. There are dozens of books reporting on today's pandemic, AIDS. There are books about possible future epidemics, like avian flu. There are "what-if" books about made-up epidemics sparked by bioterrorism. There are textbooks on epidemic malaria, SARS, dengue fever, encephalitis, HIV infection, and more. There are books about present-day epidemics of obesity, celiac disease, macular degeneration, hepatitis C, anxiety, asthma, attention-deficit/hyperactivity disorder, autism, childhood bipolar disorders, restless-leg syndrome, mind-body disorders, anger, teen sex, inflammation, methamphetamine use, terror on the Internet, absentee and permissive parents, and "affluenza." There are myriad fictional accounts of epidemics, including Defoe's *Journal of the Plague Year*, Camus's *The Plague*, Michael Crichton's *The Andromeda Strain*, and Myla Goldberg's *Wickett's Remedy*. There are dozens of films (*Outbreak*, *The Seventh Seal*, *28 Days Later*, *Panic in the Streets*, and more). The television programs, magazine articles, and Web sites on all aspects of epidemics are simply countless.

Yet amid the outpouring of words and images about epidemics, much remains hazy. There's no constant, neatly defined thing that we can all agree is an epidemic. Nor do we agree on how to describe one. For Camus, a plague outbreak in an Algerian city reveals what is most human about its residents. In Tony Kushner's *Angels in America*, the AIDS epidemic stands as a metaphor for the sickness within American society in the 1980s. An epidemic of a mysterious "leprosy" in Karel Čapek's 1937 play *The White Scourge* is a straightforward allegory of ideology-driven imperialism. Cholera reflects the fevered erotic state of Aschenbach, the main character of "Death in Venice," and the epidemic sets the stage for his demise as he yearns for an inaccessible love. These authors were not ignorant of the scientific findings on disease (by the time Mann wrote "Death in Venice," in 1912, the *Vibrio cholerae* bacterium, which causes the disease, had been known for decades, and the means by which it is transmitted were well understood). When F. W. Murnau made *Nosferatu*, the first film version of Bram Stoker's *Dracula* story, in 1922, the details of plague epidemics were well known. But Murnau made use of plague as a harrowing visual motif for the deadly havoc wrought by his film's vampire, Count Orlock. At almost the same time as Murnau was filming the plague-carrying vampire rising out of a rat-infested ship's hold to spread disease, public-health authorities were using scientific knowledge to curtail real plague epidemics in Paris and Los Angeles.

Perhaps these contrasts represent no more than instances of artistic license. Leave art aside, then. Our own reactions to illness and death reveal similar contrasts. More than 100,000 Americans die every year from unintentional injuries, including about 40,000 fatalities associated with motor-vehicle crashes. American teens and young adults are more likely to die from unintentional injuries than from any other cause; only homicide and suicide come close. Yet we don't speak about an epidemic of accidents in the United States, beyond the conversation about automobile safety—and even when we do talk about vehicle mishaps, we rarely go beyond drunk driving. By contrast, there are seven- or eightfold fewer deaths from AIDS in the United States (about 14,000 annually). Still, AIDS provides grounds for continuing admonitions about the perils of drugs and sex, as well as discussions about health-care delivery, community awareness, and sex education. Pneumonia and kidney failure are far more common causes of death, and nobody talks about those as public-health crises. What accounts for the mismatch between the human costs of disease and popular rhetoric about epidemics?

One answer is that epidemics create opportunities to convey messages. The Progressive movement of the early 1900s used epidemics as a rationale to further its program of preventing venereal disease by reshaping sexual mores. The U.S. medical establishment leaned on the epidemic message about infantile paralysis—poliomyelitis—to enable it to finance and carry out a national effort to develop a polio vaccine in the mid-twentieth century. Parents of autistic children in Britain and America today put the epidemic of autism to work to demand that vaccines not be used. Pharmaceutical companies raise the specter of epidemic cervical cancer to promote the vaccine against human papillomavirus. The nature of the epidemic message is neither clear nor constant. Often, the message seems to have less to do with the actual disease burden or death toll than political opportunism. Or money.

Sometimes the lesson we are supposed to learn from an epidemic threat is not the result of any realistic assessment of dangers, but of maneuvering by the fastest claimant or most powerful bidder. What message did "epidemic" convey when, in 2007, a man said to have "XDR" tuberculosis was arrested by federal authorities, removed from the hospital where he was in isolation, and made the subject of a press conference (and lawsuits) in the name of preventing an epidemic of TB—even though he was not infectious? What does "epidemic" signal when the World Health Organization announces that it sees a global threat in the epidemic of obesity—even though most of the people who are considered "overweight" or "obese" are less likely to die than are people who are very thin? What should we understand by "epidemic" when it is a label we can apply equally to the Black Death and restless-leg syndrome?

When officials or entrepreneurs make use of an epidemic threat to create politically or financially useful lessons, they follow a long tradition. Medieval Christians burned Jews in hopes of warding off epidemics of plague; outbreaks of cholera in the mid-nineteenth century were blamed on Irish immigrants in England and America; early-twentieth-century epidemics of plague in San Francisco and Los Angeles were said to be caused by immigrants (Chinese and Mexican, respectively); and venereal disease epidemics have been attributed historically to "loose women."

A deeper answer to the question about why hype about epidemics doesn't line up with the scale of damage has to do with fear. We humans dread death. It is only natural that the mass mortality brought by a great plague makes us afraid. And besides our dread of death, we are frightened by the prospect of social disruption. To live in civilized society is to bear a dread that goes beyond the fear of death.

Perhaps this is what we really mean when we call ourselves developed countries: we live in relative comfort for a comparatively long time (some more comfortably and longer than others, but even our poor are generally better off than most residents of the so-called developing world); we are fearful about losing this way of life. We of the developed nations seem to load epidemics with anxieties about death or the collapse of society. Sometimes we are right to be afraid of cataclysmic disease. The Black Death was a sudden catastrophe. Usually, though, nature is subtler.

The deeper answer, and the one this book explores, has to do with anxieties that go beyond the normal dread of death or destitution. To judge by our response to epidemics that are less sudden or catastrophic than the Black Death, we fear much more besides: strangers, flying things, modern technology, female sexual desire, racial difference, parenting, the food we eat, and so on. These concerns, beyond the simple dread of death, are part of our makeup. They identify us as citizens of the society we live in and distinguish our world from the ancient world of demons. The way we have responded to epidemics like polio, AIDS, and SARS, and the way we are currently responding to obesity, autism, and addiction, reveal that we bring fears to the prospect of any sort of epidemic, deadly or not.

This book looks at epidemics throughout Western history, going back to the Greeks and Romans, moving up through the Black Death and the development of epidemiology in the nineteenth century, and continuing to the present day. It looks at epidemics from three different perspectives. First, an epidemic registers as a *physical event*: there is a microbial disturbance in an ecosystem with accompanying shifts in the well-being of different human populations. An epidemic also plays a role in *social crisis*: the illness and death that spread widely act as destabilizers, disrupting the organization of classes, groups, and clans that make up the society we know. Finally, an epidemic has an identity as a *narrative* that knits its other aspects together: we tell ourselves stories about ourselves, accounts that make sense of what we see happening as well as what we fear (and hope) will happen. These three aspects of the epidemic can't be divorced from one another: all significant spread of illness also creates a social phenomenon; every social crisis moves us to make sense of it; each revision of the story of our society alters the way we study disease (and even how we define illness) and changes the pitch of social change. To read the history of epidemics is to follow a long story of the fears that go beyond the dread of death, the anxieties that make us who we are.

Epidemics often start with an outbreak of disease, but not always—and not all disease outbreaks spark us to tell an epidemic story. The so-called Spanish Flu of 1918 was the most acutely devastating outbreak of all time, with upwards of 40 million deaths worldwide in barely a year. Camouflaged by World War I, or perhaps just too catastrophic to dwell on, the flu outbreak registered hardly at all in the Western imagination, at least to judge by the absence of mention in literature or art for decades afterward. Then, in the 1970s, it became not just an epidemic but a central element of the epidemic imagination when scientists who were interested in promoting their theory that devastating flu outbreaks occur every decade or so made the 1918 outbreak an object of historical interest. Today, all discussions of flu involve some retrospection on the Spanish Flu epidemic, the rationale for "pandemic preparedness." There is an imagined epidemic that carries meanings not self-evident in the original event.

Some epidemics start without any disease being in evidence at all, as the creation of today's obesity epidemic reveals. An epidemic is a story that has different morals for different "readers": it teaches various lessons, follows differing accounts (depending on who is telling us what is happening), and can be a sounding of the alarm or a lament or an admonition. This book tells the story of epidemics—of how the way of looking at disease outbreaks affects what people see when there is one, and how, in turn, the epidemic we see changes how we act and what we fear. The story changes as society changes. As such, it has the capacity to illustrate the times in question and reveal the people themselves.

CHAPTER 1

THE SENSE OF AN EPIDEMIC

And which of the gods was it that set them on to quarrel? It was the son of Jove and Leto; for he was angry with the king and sent a pestilence upon the host to plague the people, because the son of Atreus had dishonoured Chryses his priest.

—HOMER, THE ILIAD, BOOK I

Seven years after an autumn 2001 epidemic of anthrax closed U.S. mail-sorting facilities and killed five Americans, the FBI has its man. Or so the agency claims: the master bioterrorist who spread spores and a certain amount of havoc in the tense autumn of 2001 was, the Bureau now alleges, Bruce Ivins. He was a scientist who worked on biological weapons at a U.S. government installation (we must call this "biodefense" because if the U.S. government were researching offensive biological agents, it would be violating the 1972 international convention on biological weapons). We cannot know whether Ivins was the culprit: he killed himself in July 2008, just before the FBI made its case against him public. But by now it is obvious that the anthrax scare and the years of hysteria it provoked over biological mayhem engineered by foreigners was based on a chimera.

The Axis of Evil, so-called nonstate actors like Al Qaeda, out-of-work scientists from the former Soviet Union, other supposedly nefarious outsiders and historical enemies—none of these has had a role in creating American epidemics. Besides the postal anthrax event of 2001, in which twenty-two people became sick and five died, only one other epidemic can be plausibly attributed to biological weapons in North America, a smallpox outbreak among tribes of the Ohio Valley during the French and Indian War in 1763. Neither incident was the work of enemy fighters or religious zealots. If human invention produced the two epidemics, it seems to have been perfidy by government agents: in the first case, a British military officer's "gift" of infected blankets to the tribes aligned with the enemy; in the recent one, a disgruntled scientist. The $20 billion that the United States has spent on protecting the public from epidemics created by human hands in the past decade might be pointless or might itself be putting people in danger, but in any case it has not solved an epidemic-by-bioterrorism problem, since such a problem never really existed.

The hysteria around anthrax began with an extraordinary welling up of dread. The September 11 disasters were a still-smoldering memory. The new gravity of life seemed to mute the customary talk of risk, as if organizing daily activities in order to maximize health (the low-fat diet, the buckled seat belt, the drinking of a single glass of red wine with dinner) had come to seem like self-indulgent effrontery in the face of the prospect of dying in a falling building, or as if health were simply in the hands of God or fate and not up to us. But when the bacterium *Bacillus anthracis* arrived by letter in October and people came down with anthrax, dread coalesced around the threat of an anthrax epidemic.

An industry fueled by fears of epidemics by bioterrorism existed before September 11, but it was little more than a start-up. Anthrax kicked it into high gear. As if to corroborate our fiercest anxieties, sci-fi scenarios were professed. In late October 2001, a symposium at

Harvard's School of Public Health featured estimable researchers and health officials lecturing on the possibility of crop dusters spraying pestilence. Admonitions about smallpox were heard. Pundits painted horrendous scenarios of cities wiped out by germs dropped from airplanes. Professor Walter Laqueur, chair of the International Research Council and a member of the Center for Strategic and International Studies in Washington, observed that "according to a 1980 study, spreading one ounce of anthrax spores . . . in a domed stadium could infect 60,000 to 80,000 people within an hour." The state of horror was so poignantly highlighted by the new anthrax cases that, to some, such scenarios seemed prophetic.

The Centers for Disease Control and Prevention, the federal agency charged with protecting the American public from disease threats, was unable or unwilling to define how people were contracting anthrax, who would not contract it, or what could be done to render safe those venues in which infections had occurred. The CDC is usually prompt in investigating outbreaks, but it was hampered by the FBI in this case when the Bureau insisted that some information was classified because of an "ongoing criminal investigation." Although much information was made public, almost none of it was usefully informative as to how little chance anyone ran of encountering anthrax spores, how nearly impossible it was to acquire anthrax from a person who had been infected, and how consequently minuscule the odds were that there would be a broad epidemic.

The anthrax outbreak of 2001 was an epidemic by the epidemiologist's definition, but it was an unusual provocation for panic. To an epidemiologist, an epidemic exists whenever there are more cases of a disease in a specified place during a particular period than would be expected based on experience. Tuberculosis, with 9 million new cases each year worldwide and almost 2 million deaths, is not epidemic by this standard: its toll is great, but epidemiologists have learned to expect it. Ditto malaria, which kills three-quarters of a million African children each year. Because anthrax outbreaks are extremely rare, twenty-two cases in the eastern United States in a two-month period constituted an epidemic. But there was no person-to-person transmission, and in a world that has seen AIDS, TB, and malaria, it was hardly a public-health disaster.

—m—

"Epidemic" has always been a troubled term, shifting with humankind's fears. The history of our encounters with epidemic disease is a story of people making sense of the extraordinary in terms of the ordinary. Some themes have been constant through recorded history: from malady in the ancient Middle Eastern land of Chaldea to the biblical plagues in Egypt to postal anthrax in the United States, the way we have thought about epidemics has involved ideas about place and disaster, two more-or-less concrete notions about the natural world, and a more elusive understanding of disease. For the past 2,500 years our understanding of disease has evolved with the state of knowledge about how we are affected by nature, and it has borne a changing burden of anxieties about bodies, souls, and the way we live in the world we have made. Prominently, ancient suspicions of contamination, divine punishment, and moral correction have permeated humanity's awareness of disease and continue to influence our grasp of the epidemic.

The modern use of the word "epidemic" to describe diseases was introduced by Hippocrates, the early Greek medical writer, who lived around 400 BC. In Part Three of his canonical work, *On Airs, Waters, and Places*, Hippocrates drew the first distinction between epidemic and endemic conditions:

> Pleurisies, peri-pneumonias, ardent fevers, and whatever diseases are reckoned acute, do not often occur, for such diseases are not apt to prevail where the bowels are loose. Ophthalmias occur of a humid character, but not of a serious nature, and of short duration, unless they attack epidemically from the change of the sea-

sons. And when they pass their fiftieth year, defluxions superven-
ing from the brain, render them paralytic when exposed suddenly
to strokes of the sun, or to cold. These diseases are endemic to
them, and, moreover, if any epidemic disease connected with the
change of the seasons, prevail, they are also liable to it.

Hippocrates is celebrated by modern physicians as the father of
medicine, but the significance of Hippocratic thought is neglected
by almost everyone else—most lamentably by epidemiologists and
other social scientists. His philosophical project was revolutionary;
we owe the very essence of public health to it. For centuries before
Hippocrates' time, Greeks had been attributing disease to the gods.
In proposing that illness comes from elements that can be observed
in the real world, not the acts of inscrutable deities, Hippocrates was
both amending a traditional viewpoint and reconfiguring the basic
idea of disease. His views weakened the influence exerted by human
beings' inchoate dread of the unknown, positioning disease as a
piece of the puzzle of nature—a puzzle with rules, or at least logic,
that mere humans could assess. By loosening the grip of innate
dread of the unknown, Hippocrates opened the door to investing
disease with fears and hopes grounded in the known world.

Hippocrates did not invent the word "epidemic." It predated him
by centuries. Derived from the Greek word for people or populace
(*demos*), *epidemiou* (επιδημιου) in ancient times meant to be in, or
come to, one's people: a modern English approximation might be
"having to do with being at home" or "toward home." In *The Iliad*,
Homer refers to civil war as *polemos epidemios*. The meaning evolved,
and "epidemic" eventually came to mean something like "indigenous"
or "native."

Hippocrates used "epidemic" exactly in the "native" sense, applying it to illness as part of his project to take disease out of the hands
of the gods. The Hippocratic theory of illness was that each place
had characteristic diseases. Some diseases could be related to particular environments, such as the seaside, marshes, mountains, and so

forth, and therefore were prone to establish themselves in certain places. They were "epidemic" in the sense that they were native, like the epidemic ophthalmias (inflammations of the eye) in the passage above. Hippocrates denoted as "endemic" diseases related to the "fluxes," or internal fluids, whose nature therefore corresponded to individuals, not places. Hippocrates' distinction between epidemic and endemic was not, as modern public-health textbooks claim, based on an early observation that diseases that strike occasionally but in intense episodes (epidemic) differ from those that are ever present (endemic). That was a much later development, which required a more modern consciousness.

Nor did Hippocrates connect epidemic disease to contagion. The clustering of disease was interesting to Hippocrates, since the accumulation of cases in relation to demonstrable elements of terrain and climate served his theory. For instance, he noted that what appear to be the well-known tertian and quartan fevers (those that come with a three- and four-day periodicity) of malaria occurred in proximity to marshy regions, even though two millenniums would go by before it would be known that malaria is spread by mosquitoes. His descriptions also seem to point to other recognizable conditions, such as dysentery and diphtheria. But the transmission of disease in the Hippocratic model had to do with fluxes, not invisible contagious particles.

The Greeks had inherited ancient ideas of malady as an effusion of the underworld and translated them into specific diseases resulting from explicit actions of the gods. Hippocrates' theories broke with theology. *Hippocrates made illness empirical.*

—∿—

In Homer's day, pestilence was understood as an act of the gods. The disease that decimates the Achaean army at the beginning of *The Iliad* is ignited by a flaming arrow shot by the god Apollo (the son of Jove by Leto), who is angry with the Achaean leader, Agamémnon, for his treatment of the priest Khrysês. Attributing to the gods the power to strike people ill or dead in retribution for improper acts, the ancient Greeks tried to make sense of illness and gave disease a moral meaning as well as a physical one.

The idea of pestilence as punishment lost its power with the Greeks, to be revived much later with Christianity. But even before Hippocrates' work was widely known, Greeks were moving away from the assumption that the gods were angry when pestilence struck. The historian Thucydides, roughly a contemporary of Hippocrates, saw no particular godly reprisal in the Plague of Athens of 427 BC. Writing circa 410 BC, he says:

> [The Peloponnesians and their allies] had not yet spent many days in Attica when the disease [nosos] first struck the Athenians. It is said to have broken out previously in many other places, in the region of Lemnos and elsewhere, but there was no previous record of so great a pestilence [loimos] and destruction of human life.

Making an explicit connection between disease and pestilence, Thucydides nonetheless offers only a speculation about its provenance:

> The plague is said to have come first of all from Ethiopia beyond Egypt; and from there it fell on Egypt and Libya and on much of the King's land. It struck the city of Athens suddenly. People in [the Athenian port city of] Piraeus caught it first, and so, since there were not yet any fountains there, they actually alleged that the Peloponnesians had put poison in the wells.

Thucydides' observation effectively hammers home the intensity of the plague by pointing out that it was too awesome and unprecedented to allow for theories about cause: "All speculation as to its origin and its causes, if causes can be found adequate to produce so great a disturbance, I leave to other writers." He had freed himself of the old Homeric certainties that the gods must be behind an extraordinary event. But the ordinary provided no clues as to why such a catastrophe would occur.

Pestilence remained a malleable term. Sometime before 29 BC, in the *Georgics*, Virgil invokes the word "pestilence" (*pestis* in Latin) when he reports on an outbreak of disease among cattle, *pecudum pestes*, in the Alpine regions north of the Adriatic. An agrarian treatise rather than a work of history, the *Georgics* had a practical outlook: to describe bad things that could happen to livestock if they were not managed properly. Virgil's text explicitly states that pestilence can be wholesale: "Not single victims do diseases seize, but a whole summer's fold in one stroke." But he also used "pestilence" metaphorically to indicate a scourge, a bothersome thing—like the adder he calls *pestis acerba boum*, the "sore plague" of cattle, capable of gliding under the straw that shelters the herd and harming cows with its venom. *Pestis* could point to something dire without implying what we would call an epidemic.

The distinction between "pestilence" and "plague" becomes crucial. The first implies uncertain origins without connoting punishment, while the second implies intent. From *pestis* came the French word *peste* and the German *Pest*, as well as the English word "pestilence." *Peste* and *Pest* denote a cataclysmic outbreak of disease. But in English the development was different: over time, the Latin word for delivering a blow, *plagare*, "to strike" (from the Doric Greek *plaga* [πλαγα], meaning "stroke" or "wound"), became the English word "plague." The same word, not accidentally, became the modern medical name for the disease caused by the bacterium *Yersinia pestis*, the organism that was responsible for the Black Death. Whereas German, French, and other languages that use a word derived from *pestis* to mean "plague" reflect the Virgilian era, the English "plague" connects words associated with punishment (strike, blow) inseparably to the idea of disastrous disease outbreaks.

—∽—

The connection between plague and epidemics traces to the story of Exodus in the Bible. The disasters delivered by God to the Egyptians were punishing blows. According to the text, the blows were meant to achieve an end: to get the Egyptians to free the Hebrews from slavery. The fifth plague in Exodus was livestock illness (the Hebrew is *dever*, meaning, like the Greek *loimos*, "pestilence"). That this catastrophe became not just pestilence but a plague reveals how much we need to recognize the divine intent behind the pestilence as well as the dire outcome.

Early Hebrew philosophy contributed to the understanding of epidemic disease in a different manner from that of the Greeks, and profoundly. Ancient Hebrew writing might seem to have pioneered the concept of plague as a divine blow, but Mesopotamian texts, already ancient by the time the Five Books of Moses were written down, had long before attributed disease to the work of demons. Reshaping disease around contamination was Hebrew philosophy's lasting contribution to how we see epidemics.

As with Hippocratic philosophy, Hebrew thinking was jarringly different from the traditional suspicions about possession or enchantment by dark spirits. Malaise (spiritual and therefore physical) was now the result of the specific work of a single, all-powerful God rather than various demons. But more important, malady resulted from the imprudent mingling of the pure with the impure. The Greeks also explained ailments as the intentional work of Apollo or other gods in response to human behavior rather than the unknowable whims of fickle demons and spirits. Where the Hebrews' way of thinking differed was that by focusing on contamination or pollution, judgments about disease became *empirical*.

By 500 BC, warnings against contamination passed along through oral tradition had been collected into what became the biblical book of Leviticus. There, the connections are made clear: crossing from fair to foul taints the spirit, and spiritual pollution fouls the physical body. Leviticus 7:19 reads: "The flesh that touches any contaminated thing may not be eaten." To the Hebrews, pestilence wasn't a sign of the mystifying fickleness of the spirit world but a divine work by a wrathful God insistent that humans do right. "If you behave casually with me and refuse to heed me, then I shall lay a further blow upon you. I will send a pestilence among you and you will be delivered into the hand of your enemy" (Lev. 26:21–26). Pestilence could be visited as punishment just as easily on the community as it could on the individual. In II Samuel (24:10–15), King David is given a choice of three punishments because of his pridefulness: seven years of famine for his people, three months fleeing from his enemies, or three days of plague in the land. Depending on the translation, David either chooses pestilence or merely chooses not to have to flee his enemies—but in all versions, God sends the plague. David survives, but 77,000 people die. The Hebrews thereby linked pestilential disaster to transgression and emphasized collective responsibility and shared fate. In so far as disease outbreaks come to be distinguished from other disasters, this biblical scenario, like the visitation inflicted on the Achaean host in *The Iliad*, offered an early example of disease as punishment.

The conjunction of ritual, right behavior, avoidance of divine wrath, and health is nowhere clearer than in the laws of the *kashrut*, detailed rules for eating and cooking that appear in chapter 11 of Leviticus and that are still followed by some observant Jews. Designating spiritually unclean and clean animals, the *kashrut* essentially divided the natural world based on contamination. Eating any animal that does not both have a cleft hoof and chew its cud is strictly forbidden. About twenty species of birds are unclean, among them those that famously serve as metaphors of evil in Western culture: vultures, kites, and ravens. Lizards and snakes are prohibited, too.

The Levitical laws on spiritual unease made three things clear that are important to understanding how people have come to see disease: spiritual taint has physical manifestations, it can arise without human awareness, and it can be redressed through the individual's efforts. If a person was struck by an ailment that was the consequence of contamination, it could, according to the Levitical law, be cured. Leviticus probably spends more words on a manifestation of spiritual unease, *tzara'as*, than on any other. *Tzara'at* referred to a set of three possible physical signs of a particular spiritual malaise. The three lesions were *s'eit*, *sapachat*, and *baheret*—each a different type of discolored skin. *Tzara'at* was described as visual evidence that the sufferer had committed one of a set of spiritual offenses: robbery, slander, false oaths, sexual misconduct, bloodshed, or selfishness. Some rabbis have suggested *tzara'at* represented God's punishment for a particular set of deeds, those revealing a failure to share the feelings or recognize the needs of others.

The biblical text gives complex instructions for how a priest might determine if a skin lesion was indeed evidence of *tzara'at* and how to handle a contaminated person. There is, famously, the command (Lev. 13:46) that the *metzora*, the contaminated person, dwell "outside the camp"—that he be ostracized, kept from association with the spiritually sound. And there are instructions as to how, after a suitable period of isolation whose tribulations will remind the *metzora* of the seriousness of falling off the spiritual wagon, the priests can purify him and return him to the circle of society.

Such were the ancient foundations of the modern concept of epidemic disease. Physical ailments, even if inseparable from spiritual malaise, emerged from the realm of mystery and enchantment and came to have causes that were accessible to the properly informed person. A person could avoid spiritual taint through scrupulous, self-aware control of his or her interactions with nature—in other words, humans could thrive in a universe whose underlying logic was observable in physical signs. The logic could be answered with rules, laws, limits, or codes. The instinctive human dread of chaos or the unknown could be redirected into specific fears that misbehavior, contamination, or transgression of well-defined limits would bring harm.

—◊◊◊—

At some point, the word "epidemic" appeared in Latin (*epidemia*) as a way to designate a disease outbreak. "Epidemic" was carried into Middle French (*ypidimie*) and eventually appeared in English, making its premiere in 1472, when Sir John Paston wrote that many of the English soldiers who went to fight in Brittany died of the "flluxe or other ipedemye." The progression in thought and naming was primarily a result of the tremendous outbreak of disease caused by *Y. pestis*—plague, to us—that produced astonishing and still unparalleled carnage in Europe between 1347 and 1351.

By the fourteenth century, physical disease was distinct from mental or behavioral aberrations. Diagnostic capabilities were good enough by then that physicians could be sure that these repeated visitations were manifestations of the same disease. To the survivors of those plague outbreaks, a sudden and widespread occurrence of a physical ailment wasn't a metaphor; it had quite concrete meaning. Exactly when the term "epidemic" came to be applied to the plague outbreaks isn't known, but it is clear enough that by Paston's day, everyone would have known exactly what he meant by "the flux or other epidemics."

The thinking about epidemics in that day could not be disentangled from the inchoate dread of death or randomness that had influenced the ancients, and the occurrences of plague in the fourteenth and fifteenth centuries, beginning with the first wave of the Black Death, in 1347, were still surrounded by mystery. Yet a fixed set of ideas emerged from them: disease was an identifiable, physical thing. Big outbreaks of disease had a recognizable progression in time, with a beginning, a middle, and an end. Ailments that came and went in the population (outbreak diseases, we would say today) were distinguishable from those that seemed to be around all the time, like consumption, "dropsie," "rising in the guts," or death in childbirth.

By about 1600, with plague outbreaks still a frequent occurrence in Western Europe, the defining story of the modern epidemic took full shape. By then, an epidemic was presumed to have a physical cause, not to be the meddlesome work of evil spirits or the sudden anger of a god (although the anger of the Christian God was still an important part of the story for some people). By the seventeenth century, bodily illness had become distinct from mental or spiritual maladies. Epidemics were illnesses of humans, verifiably different from animal diseases. An epidemic of common physical disorder was distinct in its origins from other events bringing widespread unhappiness, like flood or drought. And it was assumed that, eventually, the epidemic would end.

CHAPTER 2

PLAGUE:
BIRTH OF THE MODEL EPIDEMIC

> There have been as many plagues as wars in his-
> tory; yet always plagues and wars take people
> equally by surprise.
>
> — ALBERT CAMUS, *THE PLAGUE*

Plague in fourteenth-century Europe has long been the model for the epidemic. Even as humankind accumulates knowledge about coping with disastrous epidemics and becomes more self-assured about defying nature, we return to the antique memory of the Black Death. When illness threatens society, envisaging an epidemic in the form of the Black Death allows us to discharge many fears.

So it was that in the late summer of 1982, media stories reminded Americans of a link between AIDS and homosexuality with blunt and brutally insensitive headlines announcing the "gay plague." That unforgettable epithet announced our society's anxieties while commenting on American sexual politics. Pundits who spoke of the new plague as divine punishment for homosexual intercourse explicitly evoked apocalyptic scenarios.

When alarmist media used the word "plague" about AIDS, they clearly alluded to the Black Death. So does anyone who uses "plague" today. The Black Death was the greatest disease outbreak in Western history. Most historians agree that it killed at least a quarter, possibly more, of the population of Europe between 1347 and 1351—perhaps 25 million people. The Black Death was the archetypal epidemic.

Aside from being an efficient killer, plague was a cataclysm on which people piled meanings: treachery, foreignness, sanctity and faithlessness, dying for one's religion, obeying (or rebelling against) authority, and, of course, the fecklessness of nature. It acquired more layers of metaphor over time, none of which is exactly about epidemics, or even disease. We like to think that we see epidemic disease objectively today—rationally, and with a science-infused awareness. But it's debatable whether we have significantly revised our thinking since the first year of the Black Death.

In the 1980s AIDS seemed, literally, fabulous; it was reported as if it were a tale from Aesop or the Brothers Grimm. Hardly anyone questioned that the new disease was imbued with a moral. It was called a plague. Whenever we refer to something as a "plague," we mean that it is subtler than we can detect, bigger than we can imagine, a battle that we ought to be fighting but are not, or one that we are fighting but do not know it. Sometimes we mean that a threat is afoot that is capable of destroying our civilization. Or we simply signal that people ought to take things more seriously. Plague was not only significant historically as a shaping force in European civic life. It remains important in the lasting effects it has had on speech and action in the public realm.

During the plague era in Europe, which lasted from that first devastating outbreak in the mid-1300s until about 1700 (later in some parts of the continent), the template by which we interpret facts about disease outbreaks as validating our preconceived fears was forged. At the same time, public health as we know it today became a mainstay of the capacity of the state to guide the lives of its citizens.

Plague is caused by the bacterium *Yersinia pestis*. The bacterium infects rodents (rats and ground squirrels, mostly) and lagomorphs (rabbits and hares), as well as other small mammals. It enters these animals by the bite of a flea—most commonly, *Xenopsylla cheopis*, the Oriental rat flea (the species was discovered in Egypt in 1903; its name comes from Cheops, the pharaoh believed to have built the Great Pyramid at Giza).

If there are plague bacteria in an animal's bloodstream, a flea will suck them up into its stomach during feeding, after which the bacteria reproduce within the flea's digestive tract. When the flea jumps to a new animal to feed, it is unable to take in blood because the multiplying Y. *pestis* bacteria clog its feeding tube; it bites frantically, and eventually it regurgitates bacteria into the animal's bloodstream, thereby transmitting the plague organism. When rats or other hosts are unavailable, hungry fleas bite humans who happen to live around rodents and their fleas.*

For the most part, humans contract plague only through the bite of fleas that carry the bacterium. This was true even during the spread of the Black Death in medieval Europe. Once infected, humans rarely transmit the plague bacillus to other humans.** In the days before antibiotic treatment, most people who contracted plague died of it.*** Isolated plague cases continue to occur every year, mostly through

---

*The human flea, *Pulex irritans*, can carry plague, but it seems to do so only as a result of the sorts of ecological disturbances that bring humans into contact with rat fleas. In outbreaks it is *Xenopsylla cheopis* that spreads plague to humans.

**In general, human-to-human transmission happens only with a pulmonary form called pneumonic plague, in which lung infection allows the bacilli to be spread through the air to other humans via respiratory droplets.

***With the pneumonic form and another highly virulent form called septicemic (in which bacteria circulating in the bloodstream infect and grow in internal organs), most or all human cases died of the disease; the famous bubonic form, in which the bacteria produce swollen lymph glands, or "buboes," killed at least 50 percent, sometimes 80 percent, of victims.

contact with wild rodents, but they are easily treated with common antibiotics. Continuous chains of transmission from person to person, or rat to person to rat to person, are rare. Substantial outbreaks occur today only in crowded conditions under unusual circumstances. For instance, an unusually forceful earthquake in September 1993 reportedly destroyed a million homes and led to a plague outbreak centered in the Indian state of Sura that resulted in several hundred cases.

A plague epidemic is not simply an illness gone out of control: it is a natural event, one that involves many changes in the environment and whose effects resonate throughout ecosystems. A sudden outbreak of any serious disease among humans is rare. It happens only when the circumstances are aligned just so, when an improbable conjunction of climate, diet, human social arrangements, animal and insect population dynamics, and the natural movements of germs happens to occur. In effect, an epidemic is a kind of complicated accident.

THE COMING OF PLAGUE TO EUROPE

The Justinian Plague, whose first wave swept through the Mediterranean trading ports in the years 541–544, struck a region that was largely still under the sway of the Byzantine Empire (the pandemic was named after Emperor Justinian, who reigned from 529 to 565). The sixth-century historian Procopius reported its symptoms, fever and buboes in the groin and armpit followed by delirium and death within days. Plague returned beginning in the 570s and reached Rome in 589 (it was lifted the following year, according to legend, when Pope Gregory had a vision of the archangel Michael looming over the tomb of Hadrian). Subsequent salients poked as far inland as Lyon and Tours and recurred, occasionally, for two centuries. The last outbreaks occurred in the 760s.

Thereafter, no chronicler mentioned plague in Europe for almost six hundred years. When plague returned to Western Europe, it came from central Asia, passing through Constantinople, then the Sicilian port of Messina in 1347. It was able to spread through a society with newly populous cities interconnected by trade.

The reach of plague in the sixth, seventh, and eighth centuries had been constrained by the long duration of overland journeys. The incubation period of pneumonic plague (the only form that would allow for flea-free, person-to-person transmission) is very short, sometimes as little as a day, and the pneumonic form is so fatal that few plague-sick travelers on a journey of any length would have lived to infect business contacts or acquaintances in a new port of call. Overland commerce in the early Middle Ages did not involve the movement of masses of rats, as trade later would (especially once seagoing commerce in the Mediterranean connected with large caravans coming through the Near East). If animals accompanying caravans were infected with *Y. pestis*, they would likely have died before arrival, so the outbreak could not move very fast.

Europe in the mid-fourteenth century was dramatically different from what it had been in the 700s. Increased crop yields during the thirteenth century allowed for an expansion of rat populations, which would have increased the potential for animal outbreaks of plague. And the social changes that came with the waning of feudalism in the thirteenth and fourteenth centuries added to the climate changes to exert effects on humans, rats, and fleas that bumped the region out of quiescence. Some twentieth-century authors claim that the European plague epidemic began in China in 1330–1340; others put the origin in central Asia—roughly in the area north and west of India, today's Afghanistan-Turkmenistan-Uzbekistan region. Probably, plague had occurred in the central Asian high plains in the form of seasonal outbreaks for centuries before the fourteenth, flaring up when wild rodents that were carriers of the bacillus emerged from their burrows at the end of each rainy season. *Nosopsylla fasciatus*, the Northern rat flea, and other fleas that could live on rats both in the wild and in human habitations would have moved plague from its usual countryside cycle into the towns. The local rats of Asian trading centers would have carried plague-transmitting fleas to the rodents that moved with the caravans. The expansion of trade after the Crusades, linking Europe and central Asia via the Near East, created a virtual flea bridge.

In particular, trade routes linking commercial centers provided a network by which rats could migrate long distances and intermix with local animal populations. By the 1300s, European ports like Marseilles, Genoa, Naples, and Messina were well connected to central Asia via trading centers in the Near East, such as Smyrna, Constantinople (now Istanbul), and Kaffa (Feodosiya). The peripatetic rat population aboard Mediterranean and Black Sea trading ships would have come in contact with animals on central Asian caravans and picked up fleas from feral Asian rodents. Wild rodents in the high country leading up to the Himalayas were especially important, because plague might have circulated at high levels among wild mammals there.

Once in densely populated Europe, plague moved fairly quickly from town to town. It was probably the closeness of settlements, rather than the now-higher density of populations *within* Europe's fourteenth-century cities, that set the stage for the fast expansion of plague after 1347. When human settlements were isolated but not too far apart, the number of rats per human would have been high in rural dorps or isolated households. The rat-flea-human-flea-rat cycle would have spread the plague bacillus rapidly within such locales, creating sudden explosions of human plague in the countryside. Frequent travel between the no-longer-isolated rural settlements and the now-larger cities in turn helped spread plague from villages where plague was expanding rapidly but where there were few humans for it to infect to the cities, where it could spread widely among both rats and humans.

Plague's spread across the land in the 1340s was fast, but outbreaks extended erratically. After appearing in Sicily in 1347, plague had affected both Barcelona and Rome by May 1348 and Paris by June of that year—but Strasbourg, only about 250 miles from Paris, was not stricken until eight months later, in February 1349. Plague broke out in Mainz in August 1349 but not until 1350 in Rotterdam (only 212 miles away, and itself a seaport). In each place, the outbreak lasted for a year or less, although in some northern climates plague vanished for the winter but returned with warmer weather. The wave of outbreaks moved roughly clockwise along the seacoasts, from the Mediterranean northward, and from the coasts inland, then gradually eastward: the regions that are now Italy, southern France, and Spain were affected in 1348; northern France, England, southern Germany, and Austria in 1349; northern Germany and Scotland in 1350; Poland and the Baltic area in 1351; Moscow and environs in 1352. By the time it was over the population was drastically reduced almost everywhere in Europe: by the mid-1400s, after a century of plague, population had fallen by two-thirds. There were food shortages for want of labor to bring in the harvest.

Yet in its day the question of the Black Death's point of origin was not urgent. On the whole, fourteenth- and fifteenth-century chroniclers, prelates, and officials were more concerned with how plague spread and what could be done about it. In particular, European authors writing during or shortly after the first wave of plague wondered whether it was the work of God or Satan. "This is an example of the wonderful deeds and power of God," wrote ibn Khatimah in Andalusia, Spain. In Ireland, John Clyn of the Friars Minor felt the world to be "placed within the grasp of the Evil One." The communicability of plague was unquestioned in its own time, although the particular mode of communication—be it contagion, intemperate air, poisoned water, or astrological influence—was a matter of disagreement.

Pinpointing cause is a more modern concern. As plague is spread by the bite of a flea that has been feeding on an infected rat, it is the bacillus-transmitting flea bite that we now think of as plague's cause. Similarly, we say that tuberculosis is caused and spread by an airborne bacterium, carried in a droplet of sputum from a cough. We no longer wonder about devilry or divine works. Today it is *risk* we seek to uncover and predict. And by predicting, we engage in an illusion that we curtail our risk. In the fourteenth century, devilry, rather than risk, was the threat posed by outbreaks of plague.

DISEASE AND FEARS OF CONSPIRACY

To a medieval Christian, physical illness was indistinguishable from spiritual failing, and spiritual failing was the work of malign forces. The disbeliever invited the devil in. Therefore, the punishment embodied in illness might be a just desert for a failure of faith. Although the reason any individual merited the scourging wreaked by physical illness might not be self-evident, it was assumed that sickness was an expression of divine punishment for ill faith. Not yet obliged to look for causes of disease in the physical world, as we do today, Christians of the fourteenth century could see spiritual malaise behind any aberration of the body. Since physical illness was spiritual, and spiritual malaise was a flame that had to be tamped down lest it ignite a blaze of faithlessness, it was a duty of medieval Christians to prevent illness's spread. (It wasn't until much later, when physical and spiritual welfare were seen as separate, that people would decide that illness has a definable, earthly, and observable cause.)

Controlling disease, or at least curtailing the movements of spiritual distempers, required that medieval Christians act collectively. Community action taken to control the spread of plague would become public health as we know it today. At its beginnings, the motives for communal action were both practical and spiritual. An emotional tide of dread, propelled by anxiety about devilry, led people to monitor physical illness as evidence of spiritual malaise. Along with constructive actions aimed at preventing the spread of ill faith by interrupting the advance of physical disease, such anxieties about devilry led to gruesome exterminations, particularly of

Jews. The fourteenth-century Jew hunt that occurred at the height of the Black Death prefigured the Holocaust of the twentieth century and crudely illustrated how self-protection from real physical threats and dread of spiritual contamination were often knitted together in the attempt to understand plague.

For centuries before plague, fears that the bedeviled might conspire to undermine Christian society led to the exclusion of the leper—who might be anyone who was suspected, by reason of appearance or behavior, of spiritual taint. Medieval Christians interpreted very strictly the injunction in Leviticus 13:45–46 against consorting with lepers. "Being impure," the biblical text reads, the leper "shall dwell apart; his dwelling shall be outside the camp."

According to historian Sheldon Watts, when medieval Europeans followed the instructions of the Levitical text to ostracize lepers, they misidentified the disease in question. The spiritual affliction with which chapter 13 of Leviticus is entirely concerned, *tzara'at*, was not modern-day Hansen's disease (a bacterial illness).* The implication in Leviticus of barring the afflicted *metzora* from full participation in society was not that a physical illness made its sufferers unfit to be part of society. It was that the individual was expected to undertake spiritual reform. But medieval Christians, reading the

---

*When the book of Leviticus was translated into Greek, lingua franca in much of the Mediterranean basin in the third century BC, the word *lepra*, meaning "scaliness," was used to denote *tzara'at*. By rendering the spiritual term *tzara'at* with a word that merely described the outward manifestation, the translators lost the essential meaning of moral malaise. The translation error was perpetuated about six centuries later, circa AD 400, when St. Jerome compiled the Latin Vulgate. Although Jerome rejected the *Septuagint*, the Greek translation of the Old Testament, instead translating directly from the Hebrew into Latin, he simply accepted the Greek word *lepra* for *tzara'at* and adopted it into his Latin translation of Leviticus. When Hansen's disease became common in Europe, several hundred years after Jerome, it took on the name *lepre* in Old French and Middle English (*lèpre* in modern French, leprosy in English).

Latin version of Leviticus, thought that they were called upon to exile people with the disease "leprosy," i.e., Hansen's disease.

By misapplying Leviticus's injunction about moral taint to a physical condition, medieval Christians essentially created the leper.
Something essential was lost in translation. After the Council of
Lyon of 583, lepers were forbidden to associate with healthy people,
and laws regulating interactions with lepers were established. By the
twelfth century or so, a long list of characteristics could cause a person to be labeled a leper—from various skin disorders to behavior
that signaled trouble to policy makers or the church. Unlike *tzara'at*,
medieval leprosy was not redressed by a period of segregation and
contemplation. Leprosy was permanent.

Lazarettos, hostels for lepers, existed in Europe from the seventh
or eighth century, but it wasn't until the Third Lateran Council, in
1179, that all lepers were required to wear identifying insignia and
towns had to maintain lazarettos to house and feed them. Once a
specific prescription for dealing with lepers was in place, a Christian
could demonstrate his moral uprightness by giving succor to the
leper. In this way, lepers were useful to the operation of Christian society: they were scorned but cared for, and they served as a touch-
stone by which the faithful could reassure themselves of their piety.

In medieval society, people who were disdained because they had
a disfiguring disease (or were merely imagined to represent a threat)
could exist only by living apart. In this regard, the ostracizing of the
leper foreshadowed the epidemic in the modern imagination. We no
longer banish the carriers of spiritual taint, identifying them by disfigurement or skin ailments. But we do identify suspicious people by skin
color, national origin, or sexual practice today as potentially infectious. Certainly, that was the point of proposals early in the U.S.
AIDS outbreak to tattoo homosexual men and the reason for the drop
in patronage at Chinese restaurants in U.S. cities when the severe
adult respiratory syndrome (SARS) was spreading in Asia. We do not
refer to them as such, but lepers still exist in the modern imagination.

PLAGUE AND VIOLENCE TOWARD JEWS

In medieval Europe, lepers and Jews were linked in the fearful minds of many Christians. Jews, as unbelievers, were inherently "leprous." By 1215, Jews as well as lepers were ordered to wear clothing to indicate their status, so that Christians who were pure could avoid inadvertent contamination.

Like lepers, Jews might be bedeviled. But Jews were not fallen Christians, as lepers were. Nor were Jews heretics, who might seduce believers away from the "true faith" with an alternative vision of worship or different manner of obedience to God's will. Jews were suspect, but they were also valuable. Jews lent money, which made them the object of envy, scorn, and resentment. Jews prepared food differently—which might have contributed to accusations that they poisoned Christian food and drink, used human blood in rituals, or desecrated the Host. Jews were also disproportionately represented among physicians in medieval society. It might have been easy to imagine that physicians knew how to tinker with food and drink. Doctors in those days, recommending powders and poultices, must frequently have poisoned their patients inadvertently, even though their sincere intentions were to cure. Physicians were well paid and well dressed, too, which must have added resentment to suspicions cast on Jewish doctors. In a society fearful of the devil's enchantments, Jews were the cause of distress.

By the fourteenth century, fear of diabolical conspiracy largely had shifted from lepers to Jews. In 1320, the Pastoureaux, peasant youth and children rising up against the authority of the crown in France, targeted Jews, whom they saw as protégés of the monarchy. The French king demanded that Jews be protected. Yet the Pastoureaux, along with local helpers, are said to have slaughtered every Jew in southern France.

In the wake of the Pastoureaux rebellion, King Philip V of France visited Poitou in the Aquitaine in 1321, where he was told that wells

and springs had been infected with poisons by a great number of lepers (in times of distress, well poisoning had a specific resonance with
the Bible: in the Apocalypse, as prophesied in Revelation 8:1–13, after the opening of the Seventh Seal a third of the earth's waters would
be poisoned by the fallen star Wormwood). By the account of the
fourteenth-century chronicler Guillaume de Nangis, lepers were tried
for poisoning the waters throughout the region, and confessions were
extracted by torture or amid the flames while the *lépreux* were being
burned at the stake. Lepers were forced to confess that their aim was
to kill Christians or spread taint so as to turn the healthy leprous.

According to Guillaume, a nobleman at Parthenay wrote to King
Philip that one of the important lepers had confessed that a rich Jew
had encouraged him to commit the crime of well poisoning, paying
him ten pounds, with the promise of more, if he would persuade
other lepers to do the same. Jews, it was further understood, had con-
vened the principal lepers for the purposes of interventions by the
devil. "Care of the Jews, the fatal poisons were spread by lepers
through the entire kingdom of France," Guillaume wrote.

Secular authorities, who had previously supervised the maintenance of lepers and defended Jews from attacks, began to contribute
to violence against both. In June 1321, King Philip issued an edict
against lepers, followed in July by one against Jews.

When plague arrived in the region, a generation later, it served
to crystallize fears of diabolical corruption. As plague advanced and
rumors of its origin were connected to Jewish knowledge of poisons
and conspiracy to undo Christian society, a series of attacks left
Western Europe nearly devoid of Jews.

The violence against Jews began in Toulon, France, on Palm
Sunday of 1348. Just as plague arrived there, townspeople assaulted
the Jewish quarter, killing forty people. Violence against Jews during
Easter week was not unusual in that era, but subsequent events made
clear that the attacks of 1348 were a direct response to fears of the
advancing wave of plague mortality. Attacks on Jews continued in

Avignon and Grasse later that April, and spread to other towns in Provence and then Catalonia. Assaults on Jews continued through parts of Spain, the Savoy, the Vaud, the Black Forest, Bavaria (Munich, Nuremberg, Augsburg, Regensburg), Baden-Württemberg, and then the Rhineland, before moving east. Jews were accused of well poisoning, the indictment commonly leveled against suspected enchanters. With no experience of plague in human memory in the region and no focused concept of disease as the result of real-world causes, fear that the onset of plague was evidence of spiritual contamination likely motivated some of the attackers. But if so, their base fears let them be manipulated by leaders who planned to use plague for their own ends.

In Basel, mobs burned several hundred Jews in January 1349. In Strasbourg, the guilds deposed the ruling city council when it refused to persecute Jews, and elected a more compliant one. The *Bürgermeister* of Strasbourg pled for reason, but in February 1349, before plague had even reached the city, inhabitants burned the city's Jews at stakes posted in the cemetery. In March, the Jews of Worms, in the Rhineland, immolated themselves inside their houses rather than fall into the hands of the mob. In the German city of Mainz, 12,000 Jews were burned to death. By July 1349 the pogroms had reached Cologne. The last slaughters were in Antwerp and Brussels in December of that year; all the Jews of those cities were killed. Within three years of the arrival of plague in Europe, Jews had been exterminated in or hounded out of hundreds of towns and cities.

These events were not, or at least not all, spontaneous outbursts. In the case of Nuremberg, Regensburg, and Frankfurt, the Holy Roman Emperor, Charles IV, had guaranteed ahead of time that the mobs could attack Jews with impunity. In Dresden, the Duke of Meissen instructed the townspeople to attack Jews in early 1349 and promised that there would be no sanctions brought against them for doing so. Presumably, those who most believed that the outbreak expressed God's punishment, i.e., the devout poor, were easily persuaded to attack Jewish scapegoats. Meanwhile, the burghers, secular office-holders, and petty ecclesiastical officials could profit by taking over the property and valuables that Jews abandoned when they fled or died.

In some cases, there were judicial prosecutions against Jews, a sign that the attacks were not just the work of mobs aroused by private dread. In September 1348, a Jewish surgeon named Balavigny was interrogated by officials at Chillon, in Switzerland, until he was forced to "confess" that he had put into the water supply some powder that he had obtained from a "Rabbi Jacob" of Spain (a country where plague was already abroad). The *Strassburg Urkundenbuch*, the city of Strasbourg's compilation of documents, contains detail from the time on the poisons that Jews supposedly used to create plague.

The church never sought to suppress Jewry or implicate Jews in the spread of plague at the time. On the contrary, Pope Clement VI issued two edicts, in July and September of 1348, prohibiting killing and forcible conversion of Jews. He admonished Christians not to attribute plague to the Jews, accusing anyone who did so of having been seduced by the devil. As evidence that Jews were not culpable, Clement noted that Jews were themselves affected by plague. The outbreak, he contended, was the result of a "mysterious decree of God." If there was a civil conflict, then, it was between one mystery and another: God's alleged will on the one side; Jews and a recondite conspiracy on the other.

The specific charges leveled against Jews when plague loomed were recapitulations of old accusations, particularly suspicions of intentional poisoning. But the sense that poisoners threatened society had its own practical power, too: poisoning was a persistent possibility at a time when food wasn't always safe to eat; clean water might easily be contaminated by local industry; and physicians worked with apothecaries to provide patients with poultices, infusions, or electuaries (powders mixed with honey or sweet syrup) that were not fully systematized, let alone regulated. Medicines in that day were compounded of material from plants and animals or metallic substances, and treatments might have included applying plasters of dung or fumigating bedrooms with burning herbs. Chaucer, writing at the time, reminds us that fourteenth-century physicians were known to collude with apothecaries, the first prescribing medicines and the second producing them—not necessarily to the benefit of the patient but to the profit of both:

> Ful redy hadde he his apothecaries
> To sende hym drogges and his letuaries,
> For ech of hem made oother for to wynne.

With plague and poisoning commonplace, it must have been easy for people to think of the death-filled days of the Black Death as a fulfillment of the nightmare vision of Apocalypse. The sense that doom was at hand was most likely fed by a pronounced trepidation about change. Some historians believe that the militant Christianity that had held European society in thrall during the early Crusades, the so-called *Civitas Dei*, or State of God, was relaxing its hold during the century and a half before plague arrived. Certainly, with the expansion of commerce in the thirteenth century came the rise of a middle class—still affixed to the church but no longer well served by the traditional institutions of medieval Christianity. One reason for the violence against Jews might be that plague offered an excuse to take over Jewish wealth and property—a lynchpin of social tension in the thirteenth and fourteenth centuries. Had it been Christian belief alone that drove the mobs, Pope Clement's injunction would have persuaded them to desist.

It's impossible to know whether most people thought Jews had much to do with real problems of contracting disease or dying. By the time the plague's frontier had reached into northern Germany, Eastern Europe, and Scotland, the extermination of Jews was over—not because the epidemic had moved on but because the holocaust had largely succeeded in its fundamental goal: surviving Jews had either converted or moved out of the region. Attacks on Jews didn't end permanently when the plague moved to the northern and eastern regions; in the 1380s and '90s, Jews in Halle, Durkheim, and Colmar, again suspected of having poisoned wells, were attacked. Jews were expelled from Cologne in 1424 on this basis, and in 1488 a plague outbreak in Saxony was attributed to the arrival from Nuremberg of a converted Jew. So the holocaust of 1348–1349 can only have ended because the flames ran out of fuel. It might well have continued had there been Jews left to target.

Western Europe froze into deep, troubled sleep in the 1340s. The Apocalypse seemed to show itself as reports of plague and its devastation arrived, horror deepening as deaths from plague and fire piled up. There was deep-felt dread about disappearance, the imminent end of the world, and the sudden, terrible collapse featured in Revelation. Long-harbored fears about conspiracy and contamination came to focus on lepers and then on Jews (and eventually on witches). The intensity of the mortality that plague wrought was new, but the responses it elicited were, in a sense, all old news.

—∞—

With Apocalypse in mind and the dread of occult evils brought out by massive disease outbreaks, plague and penitence became inseparable. Plague offered an opportunity to confess sins and seek forgiveness. Pope Gregory had articulated the connection between plague and penitence during the Justinian plague, in the sixth century. As related by his contemporary Gregory of Tours, Pope Gregory reminded the faithful in 591 that "all the people are smitten by the sword of divine wrath; one after another they are swept away by sudden death. . . . The blow falls; the victim is snatched away before he can . . . repent. . . . Let every one of us therefore betake himself to lamentation and repentance before the blow has fallen." If pestilence is an act of God, and if the people can learn from it that the fruits of sin are disease and death, then the victims of plague give their lives for others' holy benefit.

Plague's links to sin, punishment, and salvation also became common motifs in visual art. Plague in art could be a signal of the End of Days, the primitive condition from which mortal beings could (and were expected to) lift themselves through faith, or a divine pestilence from which a city could be lifted by the intercession of a saint.

The Jesuits knew that plague could elicit repentance, and they expanded on the themes of sin and forgiveness. In the sixteenth century, some Jesuits claimed that plagues were sent expressly to purge evil and reward good. One, Guy Rouillet, called the plague outbreak in Ferrara, Italy, in 1558 an emblem of God's punishment, delivered because of divine love. Another, Everard Mercurian, wrote in 1564 that God had sent the *peste* to Tournai in order to heal its inhabitants' spiritual pestilence. The Jesuit Dominique Mengin expressed his gratitude for plague in Munich in 1562 because it turned the city's residents away from the "pleasures of this world and delights of the flesh" and toward divine sacrament. This wasn't just a Jesuit conceit; the archbishop of Cologne ordered a three-day fast and the displaying of holy relics in order to combat the plague outbreak of 1564.

To a degree, pestilence is still the context for confession. Basketball star Magic Johnson, acknowledging that he had become infected with the AIDS virus through sex, advised abstinence. Another well-known HIV-infected man, Larry Kramer, novelist, playwright, and AIDS activist, said that "we [gay men] are murdering each other. . . . I know I murdered some of them." Compared with the confessions of the time of Justinian, the modern penitent's admissions of misbehavior might be driven less by eagerness to get into heaven and more by a desire to help others through public repentance (perhaps to create a laudable public image, too). But they are confessions that would not have resounded had it not been for epidemic disease.

ILLNESS AND FAITH

Europeans' experiences throughout the period of plague outbreaks shaped the imagination of disease—and linked it to Christian faith. Depictions of plague in paintings and engravings were a kind of visual prayer, a reminder of faith. The viewer could come back to images of plague-ridden cities as she or he would come back, each day or week, to a church or a Bible reading. Disease, suffering, the lamentation of the bereaved, the vain attempts of pitiable infants to suckle at their dead mothers' breasts, the scourge of plague—all were wrapped, visually, in acts or failures of faith.

The relief of plague through acts of faith or divine love was illustrated from early on. The Limbourg brothers depicted Pope Gregory's vision of St. Michael, which reputedly lifted plague from Rome in 590, in the *Belles Heures* of the Duke de Berry in 1410, and again a few years later in the *Très Riches Heures* (see figure 1). A 1456 painting by Giovanni di Paolo, *St. Nicholas Saving Florence*, shows the eponymous saint hovering over a depopulated city while the remaining residents enact religious rites related to plague (processionals, prayer, a funeral). In Luca Giordano's *Saint Gennaro Frees Naples from the Plague* (1662), the saint hovers over a ghastly urban landscape littered with corpses, beseeching Jesus' favor. Some of the bodies show telltale buboes and others the lacerations of surgeons' fruitless attempts to save them. Faith, we are meant to understand, will save the city where earthly intervention failed.

Some plague art suggested that salvation was unattainable through holy intercession or reminded the viewer that plague was punishment. *The Piazza Mercatello During the Plague of 1656*, painted by Micco Spadaro (Domenico Gargiulo), shows a scene of Naples (the Piazza Mercatello is present-day Piazza Dante) where officials direct the cleanup of a corpse-littered landscape while the plague-stricken, dying in agony, look on (see figure 2). Gargiulo was a health deputy in Naples and must have witnessed the effects of the very outbreak that he took as his theme.

To view artwork that confirmed the connection between suffering and faith was itself a form of piety. There might be no better example of the vital power with which viewing was imbued in the plague days than Matthias Grünewald's *Isenheim Altarpiece* (see figure 3). The work was commissioned by the monastic Order of St. Anthony in Isenheim in 1505 and completed between 1512 and 1516. Grünewald created it during the period when Martin Luther, lecturing at the University of Wittenberg on the centrality of salvation through faith in God, spurred the skepticism about church practices that became the Protestant Reformation. The piece is not explicitly about plague, although St. Sebastian, who is often associated with plague, appears next to a panel showing Christ crucified. Grünewald's ostensible subject was the life, death, and entombment of Christ, but the piece had much to do with both salvation through faith and the appreciation of epidemic disease in that day.

Grünewald's altarpiece is important evidence of how physical illness was understood at the end of the Middle Ages. Illness was always pertinent to the Antonine monks. The order had been established in Europe in 1095 and named for St. Anthony of Egypt, who was said to be able to cure the illness called ergotism, or St. Anthony's fire. Ergotism results from eating cereals, especially rye, that are contaminated by the fungus *Claviceps purpurea*. It was a fairly common condition in medieval Europe. Its skin manifestations—gangrene can be one—made it distinctive at the time and led to an association with leprosy. Although the Antonines remained dedicated to curing ergotism in the Middle Ages, they were also known for the treatment of other illnesses, especially those that also caused swelling of the skin or desquamation. Thus, other conditions that would have come to the Antonine monks' attention likely included shingles, leprosy, and plague.

At Isenheim, the monks brought the sick to see Grünewald's altarpiece. The art historian Horst Ziermann makes a cogent case that the work was intended to be viewed by illiterate people, "the poorest of the poor," and thus would have been observed not from left to right, as readers instinctively do, but in the opposite direction. Meant to elicit both compassion and feelings of guilt as ways to deepen the viewer's piety, the right-to-left viewing would have taken in St. Anthony first, then the Crucifixion with Christ in obvious torment, and finally St. Sebastian pierced by arrows and draped in the brick-red cloth of martyrdom. The leftward movement of the gaze, through suffering to martyrdom and eventually to the open window, with its view of angels, was meant to engage the viewer's subconscious in pious, compassionate contemplation. It reminded the sick that their sufferings were small compared with those of Jesus and told them not only that the promise of healing was extended by St. Anthony but also that it could be read in Jesus' life. Observation was observance. The act of viewing salvation through acts of faith itself became a healing act of faith.

—⁓—

Gradually, as plague outbreaks became irregular events in Europe, plague shed some of its mystical overlay. The line between magic and medicine was still thin and easily crossed—tokens and amulets supposed to ward off disease-carrying spirits were worn well into the sixteenth century, for instance. But from the late 1500s onward, physicians made practical recommendations for preventing plague, including perfuming clothing and carrying rue, angelica, madderwort, valerian, and other herbs. In 1665 the Royal College of Physicians* published recipes that might be of use to plague-afflicted Londoners. Among many remedies offered for use internally or, in some cases, topically were instructions to drink the Plague-water of Mathias; to take Mithridates' medicine of figs or a conserve of red roses, wood sorrel, lovage, and sage; and to take a Plague-water com-

---

*The College had been established by royal charter in 1518 as a professional organization of physicians and apothecaries.

pounded of rue, rosemary, sage, sorrel, celandine, and mugwort, with brambles, balm, and other plants, steeped in white wine.

Further promoting practical responses to plague, physicians of the seventeenth century connected private cleansing with public works. The Royal College of Physicians recommended that public gatherings be banned and streets kept clean. Perhaps the repeated rounds of plague outbreaks made it obvious that everyone's chances of survival would be better if all agreed to certain collective measures.

New thinking about the possibilities for controlling plague did not displace religious devotion, but by the seventeenth century the role of the divine shared place with collective responsibility in shaping human fate. When Francis Herring of London published a monograph with rules for "This Time of Pestilentiall [sic] Contagion," he called the outbreak a "stroke of God's wrath for the sinnes of Mankinde" but also advised authorities to provide for the poor to keep them from vagabondage and to clean the streets. In Catalonia, the tanner Miquel Parets recorded both pious and practical responses to plague. Barcelona had banned trade with Tortosa, then afflicted with plague, in 1649, Parets noted. The arrival of plague in January 1651 prompted the Barcelona authorities to quarantine households struck by plague, burn the clothing of the affected, and fumigate entire streets. By April of that year, with plague continuing to spread, Parets wrote, the church had ordered that the relic of St. Severus be carried along the processional route because "our Lord was as angered with us."

Europeans of the seventeenth century might still have been enthralled by visions of apocalypse and seduced by the possibility of salvation, but many had come to observe, make connections, figure, and act in practical ways. Thinking about epidemic disease became part of *public* thinking.

PLAGUE AND THE GROWTH OF THE STATE

It wasn't until the early eighteenth century that the countries of Western Europe had a real public, in the sense that there was a realm of human affairs that represented the nonprivate doings of the many: reacting to administrative decisions by the rulers, thinking about having the state do more (or less) policing of activities in the community, exchanging news about market prices or travel conditions. But the institutions that would contribute to the evolving public nature of civil society were shaped, in no small part, by plague.

The public aspects of plague began slowly but early on, with simple measures to prevent the movement of contagion. Quarantine, the isolation of potentially infective people or cargoes, might have been used in some form or other for many years even before the Black Death, but once plague arrived it was quickly institutionalized. In March 1348, plague having settled into Venice, the doge and his council began requiring that incoming ships lie offshore for a period of weeks before entering the city proper. For a time, the duration of the holding period varied. But by 1374 it was set at forty days at Venice and subsidiary ports, based on biblical accounts giving weight to forty-day periods, such as the Flood and Christ's temptation in the wilderness. The forty-day period became customary, although it was never universal.

Venetian quarantine regulations were duplicated at Ragusa (now Dubrovnik), which belonged to Venice at the time, and adopted by Marseille in the 1480s. Later, other ports in the region followed suit. Inland cities also moved quickly to implement plague policies. Wrapping a controlled border around a town created a *cordon sanitaire*, first enacted by the Italian city of Pistoia in May 1348. Citizens of Pistoia and its *contado*, the adjoining countryside, were forbidden to travel to or from plague-stricken Pisa or Lucca except by special permission of the city's elders, while people from Pisa and Lucca were banned from Pistoia.

Eventually, use of the quarantine and *cordon sanitaire* became standard around Europe. Along the *Kaisersgrenze*, the militarized boundary separating the Austro-Hungarian Empire from the Turks and Slavs to the east, travelers crossing the *Pestkordon* from east to west after 1770 could be interned in barracks for weeks, depending on their point of origin. Goods were stored and sometimes treated with chemicals or fumigated before being released for westward transport. By providing a sense of protection against the ingress of disease, the *cordon sanitaire* contributed to people's sense of identity as a community, town, or nation. The inspection of travelers and goods became a mainstay of the idea of the national boundary, and it remains that today.

Wherever plague focused attention on aspects of the public arena, plague regulations were promulgated to accompany quarantines and cordons. By 1374, Milan had enacted laws requiring that anyone with a swelling or tumor be expelled from Milanese lands. Venice also excluded its plague sufferers, ferrying them out to islands offshore until they recovered or died. And not only plague victims were isolated: beginning in 1348, the rulers in Milan required that houses stricken by plague be walled up, isolating the entire family of the plague-stricken individual. Florence adopted the harsh Milanese regime during plague times, permitting troops to shoot individuals who tried to escape from sealed-off plague-ridden villages. London's Privy Council acted to enforce isolation on plague victims beginning in 1564; further measures were added until, by 1583, there were twenty-one plague ordinances, extending beyond isolation to include street cleaning, prohibition of public assemblies, and other programs believed to limit the spread of disease.

—⚭—

By the 1500s, a long-standing custom to mark the houses of plague victims in a distinctive manner was beginning to be made official in Western Europe. Although the sign varied, its intent was the same: the marking would warn passersby of the threat and also allow for surveillance by city officials. In 1512, the city of Rouen appointed men to paint a mark on houses contaminated by plague. Marking also became part of official edicts in Paris in November 1510 and in London and Oxford in 1518. The English laws required inhabitants of a plague-affected house to put a bundle of straw in the window (later, the mark was a red cross painted by the door) and leave the mark there for two months after the house was free of plague. They also stipulated that residents of affected households must carry a white stick whenever they left the house. The Plague Act of 1604 allowed official watchmen to use force to prevent residents of shuttered houses from leaving.

Laws mandating that plague houses be marked had a subtler practical use: they acknowledged the reach of the state into the private life of the individual while seeming to endorse the traditional religious view of epidemics. Not the church alone, or the doctrines of true faith, would determine how plague would be handled, whatever the pope might decree in his edicts or the abbots prescribe for salvation. In plague times, the two halves of civilized life joined at doorways throughout Europe, marked both so that the Angel of Death could pass by and so the authorities could corral contagion.

Taxation was less subtle than crossed doors as a reminder of the expanding role of the state in steering the public arena. Plague taxes were levied for the first time at York, England, in 1550 and at Lille, France, a few years later. After 1604, households in London could be taxed during any time of plague, and by 1665 parishes were required to collect special tax revenues from residents to support the parish pesthouse. Taking on the authority to levy special taxes in times of plague, governments turned disease outbreaks into reminders of the authority of the state in the private lives of its citizens. An epidemic became a way of solidifying a social compact: the state would defend the citizenry against disease threats but demand compliance with laws and regulations; individuals would pay taxes and give up some liberties in exchange for their rulers' and policy makers' actions on behalf of the public welfare.

When plague motivated localities to enumerate residents' deaths, beginning in the fifteenth century, it provided another important tool for the development and display of secular authority. Eyewitnesses reporting on the outbreaks of the Black Death emphasized not only the suffering but also the surprising rapidity of mortality: once plague struck, the corpses couldn't be buried as fast as they accumulated. The chroniclers Agnolo di Tura in Siena and Gabriel de Muisis in Piacenza each noted that there were too many deaths for the church bells to be tolled. In Montpellier, France, Simon de Covino observed peasants dropping dead in the fields; Henry Knighton, at Leicester Abbey in England, wrote that there were so few laborers left after plague passed through that "no one knew where to turn for help." In the diocese of Bath and Wells, many died without last rites because no priest could be found to take confession. The unusual concentration of deaths in a short period became a signal of the epidemic, and attention began to focus on the rate of death.

The first official compilation of death counts was ordered in Milan in 1452 by the magistrates who had been charged with protecting the health of the city-state. Other Italian localities began keeping similar bills of mortality shortly thereafter (Mantua in 1496, for example, and Venice in 1504). By the 1500s, some cities were keeping records of deaths even when there was no plague outbreak.

The London bills of mortality were inaugurated in 1519 by order of the corporation of London, the governing body of the city. By 1592 the mortality bills were issued even in years with no outbreak of plague. In that era, the tolling of church bells would alert women called "searchers" that a new death had occurred. The searchers would ask the parish sexton to call out matrons, who were appointed to view the corpse and make a judgment as to the cause of death. The particulars of the death were then reported to the parish clerk, who compiled the number of deaths by cause for his parish and submitted a report each week to the city's registrar of deaths. Starting in 1603, the registrar issued his bill of mortality weekly to the king. Sometime in the 1610s the mortality bills began to be published, and print copies were made available through the city. In 1629 the company of parish clerks in London expanded the bills of mortality to account for weekly deaths from all causes, replacing the previous record-keeping system that had produced only a count of total deaths and a separate category for plague mortality.

By the seventeenth century, the practice of using mortality records to discern the rise and fall of an epidemic had been formalized. John Graunt, the father of the modern discipline of biostatistics, published his *Natural and Political Observations Made upon the Bills of Mortality* in 1662. There, Graunt noted that certain conditions seemed to produce consistent mortality from year to year—the ratio of number of deaths from some diseases to the total number of deaths was roughly constant. Mortality from other diseases, plague being most notable, fluctuated. Graunt speculated that outbreaks of plague might be heralded by increases in the numbers of.deaths from "purples, small-pox, and other malignant diseases" occurring in nonplague years.

Reviewing more than twenty years' worth of weekly mortality bills, Graunt observed that a new disease, rickets, had appeared and that some women were dying of "rising of the lights," previously unseen. He could distinguish "sickly" years from healthful ones by the higher number of deaths in the former. And he observed two distinguishing characteristics of sickly years: there were epidemics of spotted fevers, smallpox, or dysentery, and fewer babies were christened (that is, the birthrate went down, apparently because illness reduced fecundity). The city's state of health depended most, he averred, on "the Accompts of Epidemical Diseases"—plague foremost among them, of course, but poxes and fluxes as well.

From the accounting of the number of deaths each week in each parish it was a small step to put the study of mortality into service for purposes of understanding how society worked. Through the detailed study of mortality patterns initiated by Graunt, epidemics came to be seen as part of the complex nature of human society.

Quantitative studies like Graunt's demonstrated what was long appreciated intuitively: when disease comes it takes root among the indigent. Samuel Pepys, the seventeenth-century London businessman and bon vivant whose diary reveals much about bourgeois life of the day, commented on the distinctive suffering of the poor. They were unable to flee the city when plague came, in 1665, he noted. Even in the time of the Black Death, people had been aware that the poor were in worse trouble than the well-to-do. Boccaccio's *Decameron* tales are told by ten patrician men and women who have been able to retreat from the onslaught of disease in Florence. Contemporary chroniclers noted that the plague preferentially struck the poor, generally sparing men of means. To study how epidemics work was, and still is, to explore how society keeps the wealthy separate from the hungry. The science of epidemiology was born of this realization. To see epidemics as a product of social arrangements, poverty in particular, was to open a new area of inquiry—and trigger a new set of anxieties.

The pesthouse was another symbol of state authority motivated by plague, and one directed to the management of the poor. Once plague outbreaks became frequent, the leprosy hospitals, the lazarettos, became pesthouses. The Venice lazaretto dates from 1423, well into the plague era.* Other Italian cities adopted the practice of using the lazaretto for sequestering and caring for plague victims. The grand Lazzaretto di San Gregorio in Milan, built in 1488, acknowledged its role as an accommodation for the poor from the moment it was designed. The rich, it was well known, would be cared for at home if plague struck, or they would flee. Pesthouses became the place of both exile and care for plague victims who were unable to flee and too poor to pay for their own care.

---

*Some historians—for instance, Brossollet and Mollaret—claim that the word "lazaret," *il lazzaretto* in its original Italian form, came from Lazarus, the patron saint of lepers; others hold that it was a corruption of *Santa Maria di Nazareth*, the name of a monastery standing on a small island off Venice, which, along with an adjoining island, became the place for seclusion and isolation of people with plague starting in 1423.

The builders of the Milanese lazaretto were aware that it was meant to be used for plague victims, not lepers, from the moment a hospital for the contagious was first discussed. The 1485 plague outbreak, said to have claimed 135,000 lives in Milan alone, pressed the project forward. Its architect, aptly named Lazzaro Palazzi, designed the building as a quadrilateral so that there would be one entire side for each grouping of inhabitants: the "suspected," the sick, the convalescent, and staff. The lazaretto in Milan saw its first major use in 1524, in the outbreak known as the Plague of Carlo V, and is said to have accommodated 16,000 persons in the great plague outbreak of 1630—apparently by expanding its capacity with temporary huts erected in the great courtyard.

Acknowledging the Lazzaretto di San Gregorio's role as an accommodation for the poor allowed the city-state of Milan both to care for its people and to police the poor. Cities around Europe followed suit.

—◊◊◊—

As plague returned every few years through the sixteenth and seventeenth centuries, the ancient and unreasoning dreads of death coexisted with a nascent public sensibility. Rationally, society continued such practical concerns as maintaining markets, defending territory, and ensuring supplies of food and potable water. State-directed mechanisms for plague response continued, too. When plague made spiritual failing seem widespread, however, paranoia (about lepers, Jews, or witches) could lead the way to devil-combating immolations or prosecutions based on accusations of poisoning. A man named Cadoz was arrested and decapitated for allegedly spreading plague-causing powders in Toulouse in 1545, several people were prosecuted for daubing plague ointments in Anvers in 1571, and two men were hanged and then burned on suspicion of fomenting the dreadful plague in Milan in 1630. Still, as much as nightmare visions associated with plague occasionally evoked such ferocity, they increasingly gave way to the public administrative arrangements, like quarantine and the pest-house, that were more sober, if not always more fair. By the sixteenth century and more so in the seventeenth, European communities acted out of subtler and fundamentally earthbound views of their society: they invented new programs and policies to control disease.

In the newly public society of Western Europe, plague offered excuses for social control as well. Sequestering people who might be contagious and goods that might be contaminated were useful commercially and politically. When the state locked up people or their salable merchandise for a few weeks, it reduced competition. It also made clear who was in power and demonstrated what could happen if the powerless got uppity. Helping to prevent the spread of plague became not merely an aspect of local authorities' good management of a town, but both a sign of the citizens' assent to self-regulation and the state's capacity to protect its own power. And it was a reminder that the wealthy and well-placed would take charge of regulating the poor.

As the public sector developed, contagion became increasingly important to economic welfare. Accordingly, governments regulated the public aspects of plague as they would commerce. Venice and Florence established special boards of health in 1348, at plague's initial visit, to oversee the administration of the plague-stricken city. At first, these ad hoc boards were empowered only during the plague period. Eventually they became official and permanent. The forerunners of modern municipal health departments, with some of the same extralegislative powers to create policy to protect public welfare, boards of health made the control of disease into a political problem—inevitably bringing the city's need to protect its health into conflict with its burghers' need to make money.

—ᔕᔕ—

When it withdrew from Europe, plague did so rather suddenly. England's last large outbreak was in 1665, the Baltic region's in 1709–1710, Vienna's in 1713, France's in 1720–1722 (in Marseille and environs). Outbreaks continued in the southern areas of Eastern Europe into the 1800s, and there were eruptions in Astrakhan as late as 1878–1879. But plague was a distant memory in Western Europe by the nineteenth century.

Why plague disappeared is a matter of debate. There were changes in living standards, certainly—in England, brick houses with stone or tile floors came to replace wooden ones with earthen floors, restricting the movements of rats. But the development of better housing was so gradual and geographically spotty that it does not sufficiently explain the sudden cessation of plague outbreaks. Quarantine and *cordons sanitaires*, whose use spread eastward, might have helped limit the movements of infected fleas and thus might have made outbreaks less frequent. But sanitary measures including quarantine and cordons had been in place in Western Europe for centuries before plague outbreaks vanished. And an important one, the great 1,900-kilometer *Pestkordon* at the Austro-Hungarian Empire's eastern border, was not completed until fifteen years after the last outbreak of plague in the region.

While human works might have played a role in reducing plague's power, it seems more likely that there were broader ecological shifts—not in climate alone, which didn't change dramatically, or in rat species, but in an intricate combination of factors. The black rat was replaced in Europe by the brown, or Norway, rat, but this shift, as much as it might have assisted in plague's decline, occurred too late to have instigated the disappearance of plague. There have been theories of sudden biologic shift, like acquisition of immunity by rats or mutation of the plague bacillus, but they simply don't hold up. Plague never disappeared worldwide—there are still isolated cases of it where there are wild rodents, and outbreaks continued in Asia into the modern age. What we can learn from such theories is that, however much we are drawn to simple causal explanations, the appearance and disappearance of epidemics is always a complicated matter. Epidemics are fickle things, impossible to forecast. If they obey laws of nature, then those laws are partly, and sometimes entirely, beyond human ken.

"BLACK DEATH"

It wasn't until the 1800s that the term *Black Death* was finally coined to name the great outbreak of the 1340s. To resort to metaphors like the Black Death is to create distance. Many people, perhaps most, can allow themselves a certain naïve optimism about life's likely continuance. We train ourselves to view war as the sudden threat to civilization's vitality but to see nature as benign. We get used to thinking of natural disaster in the form of hurricane or earthquake as a random event, taking perhaps a large toll in one locale but not everywhere at once. To face the stark reality of millions of deaths occurring in the space of a matter of months would shake our serenity and ruin the optimistic view that we inhabitants of the modern developed world hold. Metaphors allow us to preserve our illusion about nature being friendly.

We do not merely allude to the Black Death when we talk about plagues today; it is the basis for real expectations about contemporary epidemics. We presume an epidemic will have a beginning and an end. When disease doesn't stop, when it just keeps coming, we no longer refer to it as epidemic. If malaria is not considered epidemic now despite the three-quarters of a million African childhood deaths it causes every year, that is because malaria does not fit the epidemical expectation. Obesity is called an epidemic, in part, because we think we will somehow conquer it.

The Black Death is also our model for the central role of public reaction in defining an epidemic. Until there is a public response, there is no epidemic. Autism became an epidemic only once policy guidelines in the United States required that public schools make accommodations for autistic children. Attention-deficit/hyperactivity disorder acquired the "epidemic" title only after medications were marketed to treat the condition. Illnesses that summon no visible re-action in the public arena—even severe disorders like liver and kid-ney diseases, which together kill almost as many Americans each year as does the much more famous diabetes—do not fit the model. Liver and kidney diseases are never called epidemic.

The epidemic as we imagine it is marked more subtly by an am-bivalence about causes. An epidemic must be attributable to people who are disliked or activities that are disdained. In the 1340s those who believed the plague was summoned by a failure of religious alle-giance could rationalize blaming Jews. Those who thought it was brought by trade quarantined incoming goods from suspicious ports, or simply from commercial competitors. Others who imagined plague to be intentionally carried by foreigners closed the borders or even executed outsiders.

Latter-day epidemics with elusive causes allow people to lay blame. The anthrax outbreak of 2001 was like that, with "bioterror-ists" in general and, now, the late microbiologist Bruce Ivins in par-ticular said to be accountable, but the actual pathway by which rare anthrax germs made people ill is still a mystery. So was the salmo-nella outbreak of 2008, said to be caused by contaminated tomatoes and then associated with jalapeño peppers. AIDS is the main exam-ple of our day, blamed on homosexuality and, sometimes, sexual license in general. As kidney disease, Alzheimer's, and other condi-tions that are increasingly common causes of debilitation and death but are never called "epidemics" remind us, when there is nobody to blame, we do not apply the epidemic label.

Chapter 3

CHOLERA, POVERTY,
AND THE POLITICIZED EPIDEMIC

According to all appearance the cause of disease
should be found in the air, when it enters the body
in excess, or in insufficient quantity, or too much
at a time or when tainted by morbid miasmas.

—HIPPOCRATES, ON WINDS

That the air might be bad for us is an ancient suspicion. The
fevers of malaria were described as early as 2700 BC in China,
and by the time of Hippocrates, about 400 BC, they were understood
to be associated with swamps and marshes—the modern name for
the illness comes from the Italian *mal aria*, "bad air" (malaria is
spread not by the air itself but by anopheline mosquitoes that happen to be carrying malaria parasites of the genus *Plasmodium*).

Sometimes the suspicion that foul air causes illness is right—as
studies of rescue and recovery workers at Ground Zero show, material floating in the air after the World Trade Center towers fell really
did make people sick. So did the coal-dust-fouled air of London in
the mid-1900s and the radiation-bearing air over Ukraine and Be-
larus post Chernobyl. Most often, air is a vehicle onto which we
load our less definable worries.

In May 2007, for instance, the American news media were briefly but heartily preoccupied with the Airplane Man story: the U.S. Centers for Disease Control and Prevention called a press conference to announce that a young Atlanta-area attorney who had been diagnosed with tuberculosis was known to have flown to Europe and back on a series of commercial airline flights. By then, the CDC was already contacting passengers on the flights, urging them to be tested for possible TB infection. And its agents had invoked the federal quarantine statute to arrest the young man, to compel him to be isolated and treated—even though he had already, voluntarily, checked himself into a New York City hospital, where he was in isolation and under treatment. The furor was focused on the possibility that infection had spread to other passengers. CDC officials, evidently pandering to panic in hopes of justifying a new TB containment policy, raised the red flag of contagion extra high by claiming (falsely, as it turned out) that the bacterial strain with which the man was infected was what the agency was calling "XDR-TB"—meaning, allegedly, "extensively" drug-resistant but plainly implying both out of the ordinary and out of control.

The man was vilified as "grossly irresponsible" by the physician president of the International Society for Infectious Diseases; editorial writers charged the Airplane Man with the indecency of putting "his own convenience ahead of the safety of others"; bloggers called him "selfish" and accused him of "undermining . . . public health rules"; passengers on one of the flights in question filed suit against him. Predictable political overreaction followed the news. There were pronouncements by politicians about America's supposedly porous borders and, eventually, there were congressional hearings. A September 2007 report based on those hearings called into question the nation's security from foreign germs borne across borders. Airplane Man flew into a storm.

Air was at issue here, including airspace, the purity of the air we breathe in an airplane, and the rights of putatively infectious individuals to travel through the air on commercial flights. The CDC press conference, manipulating anxieties over bad air for what turned out to be political ends, was duly covered by the media (the first story was posted by the Associated Press online within minutes of the end of the press conference), and the reports focused on the risks of transmitting the scary XDR germ to air passengers. The story was created by CDC and brokered by the media as if it were about contagion, that is, but it played fundamentally on anxieties about vulnerability and the risks of modern life—worries that are behind our fear of bad air. The point was to create a political rationale for a new federal surveillance program: the agency had invented a Do Not Board program, through which the CDC would name travelers who allegedly constitute a communicable-disease threat and demand that commercial airlines not permit them to fly. It is still in effect. The new Do Not Board program went into practice two days after the Airplane Man press conference but was not announced to the public for over a year.

Tuberculosis indeed spreads by air. The germ, *Mycobacterium tuberculosis*, can float in droplets of sputum and, under the right circumstances, will take root in the lungs of a person who inhales just a few particles. And TB remains a serious public-health concern, although not so much in the developed world. Out of the 1.6 million TB deaths worldwide in 2005, fewer than 700 were in the United States (less than 0.03 percent of all U.S. deaths), only 815 in France, 849 in the United Kingdom, and 595 in Germany. TB is still a blight on the world's poor places, where crowded conditions and poor nutrition promote the spread of *M. tuberculosis* and straitened budgets won't allow officials to provide the effective preventive medications to ensure that those who are infected do not become sick.*

---

*While only a few thousand Western Europeans and a few hundred Americans die of TB each year, there are more than 500,000 deaths from the disease in Africa annually and more than 300,000 deaths in India.

But the Airplane Man event took place in the affluent world, where TB has been thoroughly controlled (since the early 1950s, American TB mortality has fallen from 20,000 deaths annually to the present low level). The man's sputum had been tested repeatedly before his trip, so CDC officials already knew it contained no detectable infectious TB bacteria—making him about five times *less* likely to transmit TB infection to others than would a person with detectable bacteria. The man had been told he wasn't infectious. He had been asked not to travel but apparently had never been instructed that it would be harmful to him or others. The man's wife, who traveled with him and shared rooms with him, remained uninfected. Importantly, airplane cabins are not conducive to transmission of TB bacilli, because of air filtration and high-frequency circulation.

The Airplane Man case had nothing to do with the real possibility of contagion. The problem in the Airplane Man episode was not TB. It was not infectivity (since the CDC knew that there was a negligible chance of that). The problem was that people fret about air and it is easy to make use of that fretting.

How the possibility of disease transmission came to be used for political gain is a story that reaches back to the early days of plague, when officials could seek backing from a fearful public for measures like quarantine or special taxes. But it really took shape during an unusual conjunction of economic development, political change, and epidemic disease—the cholera outbreaks of the mid-nineteenth century.

From its debut in the Western world in the early nineteenth century, cholera was entangled with colonial politics, industrialization, and poverty. Cholera, indigenous to the Indian subcontinent, had circulated there for centuries before the rest of the world knew about it. A global epidemic—a pandemic, in epidemiologists' jargon—brought cholera to the world's attention starting in 1817. British colonial policies had much to do with cholera's going global, and those policies were themselves tied to industrialization in Britain and movements in the economy and society that were linked, in turn, with utilitarian social policies. When cholera reached the British Isles and proved to wreak its worst harm among the poor, supporters of utilitarian policy invoked cholera's toll as rationale for both refurbishing urban infrastructure and holding the poor responsible for their plight. When it reached North America, cholera seemed to validate suspicions that cities in general and the impiety of the urban poor in particular were America's main social problems and the culprits in spreading epidemics. Key to this complex interrelation of policy and illness was the contention that cholera was spread by airborne clouds of decayed organic matter—miasmas.

Cholera occurs when a person ingests water or food that is contaminated with human feces containing the *Vibrio cholerae* bacteria and a large population of the bacteria enter the lumen of the intestine (i.e., the space in the center of the intestinal tube). The bacteria multiply, covering the inner wall of the intestine. There, the *V. cholerae* give off a toxin that enters the cells lining the lumen. Once inside the cells, the toxin disrupts molecular systems that are responsible for transport of salts and water across cell membranes to and from the intestinal lumen. As a result, water begins flowing out of body tissues via the intestines. The sufferer suddenly experiences profuse watery diarrhea, losing up to 30 percent of body weight. He becomes dehydrated and within a few hours enters acidosis. Untreated, cholera kills about half of the people who contract it, with death occurring from shock, kidney failure, or heart failure; those who survive acquire some immunity. Alive or dead, the victim will have excreted millions of *V. cholerae* organisms before the siege has passed, and if those bacteria find their way into the water supply or onto the hands of other people that then go into their mouths, further cases will occur. Cholera bacteria can even be carried in the intestines of people who do not get sick and who unwittingly pass the vibrios along to others.

Nowadays, cholera is treatable (simply by reversing the pathology: administering large quantities of water and physiological salts by mouth, so-called oral rehydration therapy, developed in India in the 1960s). But before treatment was established, cholera was both deadly and intractable.

CHOLERA'S BEGINNINGS

Cholera had probably circulated continuously on the Indian subcontinent for many centuries, but it was unknown in Europe or the Americas before the 1800s. Until the British entered India in the mid-1700s, cholera could have survived at a constant low level by traveling from river settlements out to the hinterlands and back as crowds moved to and from festivals. It likely resided more or less permanently in contaminated waterways, causing disease intermittently among the young but probably not much among those who survived childhood, essentially recycling itself in a persistent equilibrium. New pilgrimages or the arrival of new holiday celebrants could have provided fresh batches of susceptible young people for cholera bacteria, but with acquired resistance and an inconstant source of vulnerable bodies, transmission would have stayed low. In turn, the minimal transmissibility of V. *cholerae* would have kept its virulence relatively low.*

Also, since the subcontinent was heavily forested and relatively underpopulated, villages were mobile communities that relocated to more productive or healthier sites if the rains failed or disease broke out. Thus, cholera would have been a relatively mild, intermittent, and local phenomenon, not a cause of sudden, severe, or widespread outbreaks.

---

*A virulent microbe has poor evolutionary chances except when transmission is very common. Since the most aggressive microbes tend to kill the people they infect before they can be passed along to others, the most virulent strains are less likely than milder ones to survive.

By the late eighteenth century, the cholera vibrio had become a habitué of battlefields on the subcontinent, profiting from unsanitary conditions and the movements of masses of people. Such masses included refugees evicted from their villages by war and large companies of camp followers who, once the British East India Company arrived, were encouraged to travel with troops. It was only after the Company took control of Bengal, in 1757, that cholera had a chance to become broadly epidemic. By implementing price controls on food supplies, the Company constrained local grain transfers to maximize its profits. When drought arrived in the region in 1769, the Company's limitations on rice shipment helped produce widespread famine. It is estimated that 10 million Bengalis died in the famine period of 1769–1770.

Disease was the inevitable accompaniment to famine and displacement. Cholera was suddenly widespread. The first subcontinent-wide outbreak of cholera took place in 1817. It presaged the debut of cholera in the West, where disease outbreaks would be of an intensity not experienced since the plague years.

How exactly cholera left India for parts west after 1817 isn't clear, but it surely involved trade. The vibrio can live for days in water tanks, such as those that ships would have carried, and presumably it can survive even longer in the water stored in a camel's hump—allowing for the bacterium to move eastward to China and Japan and westward to the Arabian Peninsula by ship between 1820 and 1822, and into Afghanistan and Persia along caravan routes. After cholera was carried to Muscat, at the northeastern end of Arabia, in 1821 by British troops who had presumably picked it up in India or Afghanistan, an outbreak there allowed for further dispersion into northeastern Africa via the Arabian slave trade. By the mid-1820s, another salient of cholera's advance had reached as far north as the Caspian Sea; Russian troops returning from military campaigns against Persia and Turkey between 1826 and 1829 carried the disease north to Moscow; Russian suppression of the Polish revolt of 1830–1831 brought it to the Baltic littoral and Warsaw; thence it spread westward, entering England (1831), France (1832), and the United States (1832).

A DISEASE OF THE POOR

Cholera brought a wave of death to Europe. Hungary lost 100,000 people when it swept through in 1831–1832. Hamburg and the other Hanseatic ports were hard hit. The poorest cities, and the poorest parts of any city, suffered most. Historians report that one-eighth of the population of Cairo died of cholera in its first outbreak, in 1831. In July 1832, dozens of New Yorkers were dying each day of cholera—mostly the poor, because the more affluent New Yorkers, apprised of cholera's advance across the Atlantic, had already fled. In the summer of 1832, 95 percent of cholera decedents in New York and 90 percent in Richmond, Virginia, were laid to rest in paupers' graves.

The first cholera outbreak in England began in the fall of 1831, after a ship from Hamburg docked at Sunderland, on the northeastern coast. Cholera arrived in London the following February. By the end of 1832, the registrar's office had recorded more than 31,000 British cholera deaths, amounting to about three out of every thousand residents of England, Scotland, and Wales. But in London, with more people living on each acre of land and thus, in the absence of adequate sanitation, effectively sharing one another's waste, it was worse: roughly 1 percent of the population of London died of cholera, ten out of every thousand, three times the British average. About 5,000 Londoners died in a matter of months. Cholera's toll on the poor highlighted the excesses of the Industrial Revolution in Britain, especially in the fast-growing and overcrowded cities of England. The plight of the destitute became a main feature of public discussion, marked by ambivalence about how much help to offer them. "Improvident habits are the ruin of the labouring classes. Idleness, drunkenness, and waste, bring woful [sic] want," wrote the chaplain of poorhouses in the area of Bath in 1837.

Beginning in the late eighteenth century, British cities hypertrophied as industrialization demanded more and more cheap labor. The population of Leeds more than doubled between 1801 and 1831. London's population, also increasing more than twofold between 1801 and 1841, reached 2 million. By 1861, a quarter of the population of Britain resided in just six cities. This dramatic urbanization was abetted when the English system for poor relief was revised to drive rural subsistence farmers and cottage workers off the land and into the factories. By 1841, roughly 70 percent of the population of Liverpool consisted of laborers—which included children as young as six or seven years of age. The preponderance of the urban poor lived in appalling squalor. Sanitation was sorely lacking, especially in workers' housing, which was hastily and cheaply built by the labor-hungry factory owners. In one laboring-class district in Manchester in the 1840s, 7,000 people had no regular sanitary facility—not even a privy—other than thirty-three large chamber pots that had to be carried through the living quarters and emptied into the street each morning.

The prevalence of destitution became obvious, and the abominable living conditions of the poor were plain to the eye and the nose. In *Hard Times* (1854), Charles Dickens describes "interminable serpents of smoke" that "trailed themselves for ever and ever, and never got uncoiled" in the air of a Midlands industrial city. In her 1848 novel, *Mary Barton*, Elizabeth Gaskell describes an urban scene in Manchester:

> Berry Street . . . was unpaved; and down the middle a gutter forced its way, every now and then forming pools in the holes with which the street abounded. Never was the old Edinburgh cry of "Gardez l'eau!" more necessary than in this street. As they passed, women from their doors tossed household slops of *every* description into the gutter; they ran into the next pool, which overflowed and stagnated. Heaps of ashes were the stepping-stones, on which the passer-by, who cared in the least for cleanliness, took care not to

put his foot. . . . You went down one step even from the foul area
into the cellar in which a family of human beings lived. It was very
dark inside. . . . The smell was so fetid as almost to knock the two
men down.

No longer were the indigent vaguely pitiable hayseeds to the
upper and middle classes, as in more agrarian times. As the urban
proletariat swelled and became noisome, poverty became threatening.
The very existence of a tremendous population of the indigent was a
rebuke to smug assumptions that the modern industrial state could
take care of all its citizens, but the heavy burden of communicable illness that the laboring classes lived with and died from made the poor
both distasteful and fearsome. As industrialization continued, the
vast, dense cloud of the destitute became highly mobile as they wan-
dered in search of low-wage work, always at the mercy of business cycles (the least skilled would be the first laid off when profits shrank),
crowding into airless and squalid dwellings covered in grime and filth.
It was a perfect recipe for spreading contagion. Cholera was the worst
but not the only scourge of impoverished urban laborers, especially
in England. Typhoid, diphtheria, typhus, smallpox, and tuberculosis
were common, and mortality was high, particularly among slum
dwellers.

Friedrich Engels, the son of a factory owner, sensed the dissolution of human lives in the foul-smelling Midlands towns, so much so
that he was moved to publish *The Condition of the Working Class in
England* in 1844. In it, Engels reported that a fifth of the population
of Liverpool, more than 45,000 people, were crowded into 7,862
"damp, badly ventilated cellar dwellings," amounting to more than
five to a room; in Bristol, 46 percent of poor families were living in a
single room each; in Nottingham, about three-quarters of the houses
were built back-to-back, so that "no through ventilation is possible,
a single privy usually serv[ing] four houses." He recounted similar
horrifying conditions in industrialized cities and towns throughout

the British Isles, decrying also the alcoholism, abandonment, and prostitution that seemed to him the unavoidable accompaniment to the degradation of workers and their families.

When Karl Marx and Engels wrote, in the *Manifesto of the Communist Party*, "All that is solid melts into air, all that is holy is profaned, and man is at last compelled to face with sober senses, his real conditions of life," they gestured toward exactly the foul-smelling air of the cities where the laboring classes were packed. The domination of society in industrializing lands (including not only England and Scotland but Prussia and parts of France) by the machinery of capitalism and the machinations by which owners enriched themselves transformed air into something almost palpably foul and disease-generating.

THE POLITICAL TRANSFORMATION OF ILLNESS

For critics of industrial capitalism, the living conditions of the poor, including their ill health, were evidence of the inhuman force of capitalism. To supporters of the industrial state, contagion signaled not capitalism's excess but its vulnerability. Cholera, typhus, and the other diseases of the indigent endangered the growing economy— and thus the stability of middle-class society. Taking advantage of the new asperity toward the poor, the champions of industrialism transformed disease into a *cause* of poverty. To prevent the communication of illness would be to alleviate the weighty burden that indigence placed on the state. In the process, the "deserving poor" would come to light—with their health improved, they would work more productively. On the other side of the coin, the ones who remained poor—who could be presumed to be lazy, shiftless, or just beyond help—would be *forced* into productivity. In Britain, the foundation of this transformation was reform of the Poor Laws. The keystone was the embracing of a new view of contagion by which clouds of vapor given off by decayed organic matter, so-called miasmas, were held to spread disease.

England's Poor Laws, outlining the standards and procedures by which the destitute would receive relief, dated from 1601, and Scotland's dated from 1579. Prompted by the need to make arrangements for maintaining the victims of plague and their families, the old Poor Laws had held each parish responsible for caring for its own indigent (the English law also allowed local magistrates to levy taxes to do so). A 1662 addition, the Act of Settlement and Removal, had limited paupers' source of support to their home parish, so that they could not take advantage of differences in largesse from place to place. Workhouses were established by localities aiming to relieve their burden by concentrating the poor and making use of their labor, the first workhouse opening at Bristol in 1696. But by the nineteenth century, with economic distress both deeper and further reaching, the cost of sustenance for Britain's poor had become unsupportable (it was estimated to have climbed to 7 million pounds sterling by 1832). The curtailment of movement created by the old laws also made it more difficult for manufacturing concerns to recruit sufficient labor to increase productivity. Reform was mandated by the needs of the industrial machine. Accordingly, the broadest aim of the New Poor Law of 1834 was to free the British labor market to promote profit making by factory owners.

The new law denied poor relief to able-bodied men outside of strictly regulated workhouses, where they would be forced to contribute to the economy and maintained on an austere regimen. One of the guardians of the workhouse at Bridgwater detailed the diseases contracted by its residents in the 1830s, including measles, TB, marasmus, and diarrhea, which he attributed to the gruel-and-water diet. He pointed out that convicts at the Mill Bank penitentiary were also "gruelled into diarrhea or dysentery," and wondered why the poor should be punished as harshly as the felons were. By heaping indignity on the indigent, the New Poor Law allowed the affluent to deflect onto the poor the fears they harbored of the potential for disaster to disrupt their comfortable lives.

Edwin Chadwick, the architect of Poor Law reform, made con-trol of disease outbreaks central to the question of poor relief. Work-ing his way up to head of the Royal Commission charged with investigating the laws, Chadwick (with the economist Nassau Se-nior) had written the crucial Poor Law Report in 1832, in which he pressed for centralization of relief and promoted the use of coercion to force the poor into the workforce. He advocated reform of the old relief system in part out of the customary belief that, by making aid to the poor more efficient, Britain could reduce the costs of sustain-ing the destitute in the short term. But Chadwick was an acquain-tance of physicians Thomas Southwood Smith, Neil Arnott, and James Kay-Shuttleworth, and he was swayed by their conviction that disease contributed to destitution. In the opinion of these San-itarians, and ultimately in Chadwick's view, sanitary projects would allow government to maintain a lowered tax burden and reduce the size of the population of poor people who had to be sustained. Therefore, Chadwick also wanted disease-prevention programs to be part of a long-term solution to the problem of poverty.

A cholera outbreak in 1848–1849, even more severe than that of 1831–1832, galvanized the British parliament to act to control dis-ease. Some 15,000 Londoners died in this second cholera outbreak (more than 0.5 percent of its population of about 2.5 million—the equivalent of 43,000 deaths in today's London). More than three hundred people died each day in the first week of September 1849.

The new cholera outbreak was clearly associated with water from the river Thames, as demonstrated by physician John Snow in one of the early examples of epidemiologic investigation.* Snow's finding

---

*Snow compared the cholera death rates among households whose drinking water was drawn from the Thames below London (thus containing the city's sewage) with the mortality in households whose water came from the upper Thames or elsewhere. He found a far higher cholera death rate in families that were drinking water containing London's waste.

might seem intuitive now, but it was not in its own day. Although it was widely agreed that cholera was contagious, the Sanitarians were preoccupied with London's air, not its water. By the cholera era, most educated people were aware that disease was transmissible and fixed on air as a likely vehicle for the contagion. Miasmas were thus the focus of suspicion as the culprits in nineteenth-century cholera epidemics.

Consequently, a primary project for the Sanitarians was the elimination of miasmas from the city. As head of the newly formed Metropolitan (London) Board of Health, Chadwick's attempt to eliminate the foul odors emanating from accumulating waste led to the Nuisances Removal and Contagious Diseases Prevention Act of 1848. Since some of the companies supplying drinking water to the city's residents took their water from the Thames, as Snow knew, the extensive pollution of the river with feces resulting from compliance with the Nuisances Act might actually have helped spread cholera. But had there been no Nuisances Act, the state of London's water supplies would have made cholera transmission nearly inevitable anyway.

Chadwick's advocacy for sanitary measures as both a public good and a duty of the state was influential in Britain. Sanitarianism spurred the formation of a Commission on the Health of Towns, which proposed that Parliament enact legislation to improve housing and sanitation in the name of disease prevention. Although Parliament was slow to legislate sweeping changes in living conditions, it did enact more limited laws giving some agencies the authority to upgrade housing in the name of health. The state had long before taken on the responsibility for improving public health through measures to control disease, like quarantine. With cholera as a reminder that the lower classes, whose labor fueled the industrial engines on which the might of the British government was based, were vulnerable to unpredictable acts of nature like cholera, Chadwick's Sanitarianism burdened the state with the weighty responsibility of improving the welfare of the poor to render the whole population less susceptible.

Chadwick's brilliance was in intuiting how to use epidemics for political ends, casting blame without explicitly holding anyone accountable. The awful cholera outbreak of 1831–1832 redefined feelings toward the poor just at the moment that poverty was beginning to be visible in industrializing cities. Chadwick understood that when his countrymen felt sympathy for the poor or shame at the terrible living conditions of the destitute, they were also horrified and fearful. The cholera outbreak of 1848–1849 crystallized the tension between sympathy for and terror of the destitute. By reading in the cholera epidemics a story that emphasized the need to control disease on behalf of the poor, Chadwick could promote his theory that it is disease, not the structure of the industrial economy, that makes people poor.

MIASMA AND THE RISE OF SCIENCE

Belief that foul air was responsible for disease was crucial to the Sanitarians' campaign. The awful smells of European cities had come to symbolize both economic development and the disjunction between modern urban life and the more "natural" life of the countryside. Purity of air became a persistent cultural theme. With developments in science, air was increasingly understood to be not just a neutral surround but a *thing*. Ubiquitous and indispensable, air was readily suffused with misgivings about the new arrangements of society that developed after the end of feudalism, the rise of mercantile trading states, and finally the development of industrialized nations.

In 1605, the Englishman Sir Francis Bacon argued in *The Advancement of Learning* that the five senses give humans sufficient capacity to acquire reliable knowledge of the world. By 1620, he had worked out the basics of inductive reasoning and saw how it might be used. "There are and can be only two ways of searching into and discovering the truth," Bacon wrote. "The one flies from the senses and particulars to the most general axioms . . . this way is now in fashion. The other derives axioms from the senses and particulars, rising by a gradual and unbroken ascent, so that it arrives at the most general axioms last of all." Bacon's work marked a departure from religiously inflected philosophy, emphasizing the centrality of human experience, not divine wisdom, in determining truth.

The seventeenth-century inquiry into the relation of human senses and the natural world had much to do with air from early on. The philosopher Thomas Hobbes went so far as to deny the existence of a spiritual soul—and in *Leviathan* (1651), he claimed that what religious thinkers referred to as the soul was in reality a physical entity: breath, the indispensable but in no way spiritual principle of the body. Air, he wrote, "and many other things are bodies, though not flesh and bone."

Hobbes took issue with experiment as an approach to understanding nature, but experiment nonetheless became a leading approach for natural philosophers of his time. The Royal Society of London, founded in 1660 and chartered by Charles II two years later, was dedicated to the establishment of truth through experiment and became its main proponent. From the outset, the Royal Society was concerned with the nature of air. One of its charter members, the Irish chemist and physicist Robert Boyle, conducted experiments with the then-new air pump in the late 1650s to demonstrate air pressure. The late historian Roy Porter saw the seventeenth-century natural philosophers' project on air as an attempt to bring the spirit, whose presence in the air was by then assumed to be confirmed by Boyle's pressure experiments, under experimental control.

In keeping with the new empiricism, physicians of the time began to distinguish one ailment from another through reproducible descriptions of the illnesses they saw. Among the epidemic diseases, they differentiated an illness called the sweating sickness, whose virulent outbursts were first described by the Englishman John Caius in 1552, from plague. In 1553, the Sicilian physician Giovanni Filippo Ingrassias explained how to distinguish between two spotted fevers, measles and scarlet fever. The Veronese physician Girolamo Fracastoro described typhus, a common scourge of armies and prisoners, in his 1546 text, *De Contagione et Contagiosis Morbis*. In a society

whose welfare was increasingly tied to worldly pursuits and the con-
quest of nature, these abilities gave doctors a valuable role. In 1518,
Henry VIII of England chartered the College of Physicians, later the
Royal College of Physicians.

The influence of air on disease, a focus of natural philosophy
since Hippocrates, helped shape both the evolution of rationalism
and the realm of public welfare. Royal proclamations by James I of
England in the first years of the seventeenth century restricted
stench-producing industries in London as "no small cause of the
breeding and nourishing of the plague." By 1630, the Royal College
of Physicians had foreshadowed Chadwick's Nuisances Act by recommending that those businesses that created noisome smells, including tanneries and slaughterhouses, be evicted from London.
These concerns were part of the general reaction to the stink of large
cities (London's population had reached a half-million by 1660):
Hugh Peter returned to England from exile in Holland to become
chaplain of Cromwell's New Model Army, and he took note that the
foul conditions of the streets in British cities made it hard to keep
households clean (at least by comparison with those of the Dutch).
James Howel noted the presence of animal manure in London's
streets, although he still found the city to be less odiferous than Paris,
which "may be smelt ten miles off." In 1652, London diarist John
Evelyn visited Paris, finding the Seine to be less sweet than the
Thames but approving of the air:

> [T]he incomparable Aire of Paris is that which fortifies the in-
> habitants: so that very seldom hath a Plague or other Epidemical
> Contagion made here that havock and lamentable devastation,
> which it so frequently doth in our putrified climate, and acciden-
> tally suffocated City: contrary to that Vulgar (but most false)
> Tradition, which I find in every mans [sic] mouth; that the Pesti-
> lence is never out of Paris: but this (besides the siccity [i.e., dry-
> ness] of the aire) many Naturalists ascribe to the over sulphurous
> exhalations of the streets.

The stench only worsened as the cities grew, as Engels, Gaskell, Dickens, and other writers of the day remind us. Even as it became clear that air was not just a neutral surround readily infused with harmful vapors or bad spirit, and as the view became popular that malady resulted from the work of communicable particles, the capacity of bad air to cause disease remained a powerful and beguiling idea. Describing plague in London, Daniel Defoe's narrator in A *Journal of the Plague Year* (1722) says that the epidemic was spread by "some certain streams or fumes, which the physicians call effluvia, by the breath, or by the sweat, or by the stench of the sores of the sick persons, or some other way." The London apothecary William Boghurst, also writing about plague, attributed it to "the wind blowing westward so long together." After five weeks of plague in 1665, Samuel Pepys, the London businessman and man about town, wrote that he had seen a few houses in Drury Lane marked with a red cross and shuttered, with the fearsome "Lord Have Mercy Upon Us" inscribed on the doorways, and in reaction had gone to buy some tobacco to smell—the scent of tobacco being rumored in that day to ward off plague.

—m—

In this milieu of testing predictions through observation, explicit theories of disease spread finally began to be propounded.* By the late 1600s, the ancient corpuscular theory of contagion, by which the disease-carrying airs were understood to bear invisible atoms of illness, had been revivified. Plague doctors equipped themselves with masks to keep out the vapors exuded by the sick (see figure 4). The corpuscular theory rationalized a separation of the sick and the suspected, on one

---

*Fracastoro had proposed that certain illnesses are transmitted by invisible particles in 1546, but before the microscope it would have been impossible to test his theory or even to envisage what it meant.

side, and the susceptible, on the other; and it allowed the state, rather than the church, to regulate that separation. The New Theory of Consumption, proposed by the Englishman Benjamin Marten in 1720, claimed that animalcules of the sort made evident by van Leeuwenhoek's microscope could release some sort of poison that made people sick. Marten's disciples, including the American clergymen Cotton Mather and Benjamin Colman, held that airborne animalcules caused smallpox by entering the body through the nostrils and throat when a person breathes, then releasing a "venom" that produced the disease. This theory of biological causation of smallpox was the grounds for Mather's and Colman's advocacy of "variolation," an early form of immunization that involved scratching the skin and rubbing into it some tissue taken from a person who had had the mild form of smallpox, variola minor. Sometimes variolation caused disease in the recipient, but more often it prevented it.* Hermann Boerhaave, a Dutch proponent of corpuscular disease, thought that invisible particles might remain in the body after recovery from illness, explaining why those who recover from smallpox do not contract the disease again. The London physician Richard Mead published his *Discourse on the Plague* in 1720, theorizing that pestilential contagion is propagated by air, sick people, and goods transported from "infected" places—which would have explained why quarantine could be effective.

Thus by the 1800s, theories about contagion were beginning to have political value. The utilitarian view, popular by then, cemented this link. It held that hazards to the general public should be abated for the good of all, even if doing so requires some suffering for the few. The utilitarians' approach to cholera gave rise directly to the Sanitarians' project to use contagion, and suspicions about air as the vehicle of contagion, to control the poor.

---

*The process of vaccination against smallpox that went into general use was discovered in 1796 by Edward Jenner.

Utilitarianism began as a legal doctrine grounded in a rationalist approach to society. Furthering the break with the churches that the Enlightenment had brought, the Englishman Jeremy Bentham proposed that law should promote the maximizing of happiness for the greatest number of people. Equating happiness with the accomplishment of pleasure and avoidance of pain, he postulated a "felicific calculus" by which competing possibilities could be assessed according to the sum or pleasure or pain they produced.

CHOLERA AND UTILITARIANISM

Cholera and utilitarianism were curiously allied. Bentham's disciple, James Mill, published a six-volume history of India in which he claimed that Indian society had been essentially static since ancient times (against all evidence, and without having ever visited the subcontinent), thus justifying British conquest and dominance over its people. Mill's writing allowed him to become an official of the British East India Company in 1819; he rose to head its office, located at India House in London, just before cholera made its first appearance in the city.

Utilitarianism's place in the shaping of epidemic thinking went much beyond India House, though. John Stuart Mill, the son of James Mill, injected virtue into Bentham's felicific calculus. For Mill, moral good derived from the increase of happiness, and he asserted that what mattered was the average happiness of society's members. By Mill's logic, diminishing the threat to the general public posed by a disease like cholera would outweigh a very few citizens' intense discontent when Sanitarians forced them from their homes for the sake of sewer installation or cesspool drainage. The felicific calculus replaced the old moralism of the churches with a new moralism about achieving substantive ends. And in a society that staked its welfare on the success of industrial capitalism, it was the enlightened and affluent classes that would decide which ends were desirable. Mill was a great proponent of liberty but was skeptical about extending rights

too widely: as the historian Sheldon Watts has pointed out, the subject peoples in Britain's colonies were not guaranteed the liberty Mill
demanded for British citizens. "Despotism is a legitimate mode of
government in dealing with barbarians," Mill wrote. "[T]here is nothing for them but implicit obedience to an Akbar or a Charlemagne, if
they are so fortunate as to find one."

With Mill's form of utilitarianism the liberals could reassure
themselves they were helping the laboring classes, the colonies, and
the impoverished unemployed. The powerful extended a hand to
the poor but demanded in return that the poor toil in the economic
engine that helped the industrialists grow rich. Thus, the austere
workhouses of the New Poor Law were readily rationalized. The
state would offer considerable access to liberty and the goods that a
growing economy can offer, but for that the pauper had to donate
her labor to produce capital. If the poor didn't join the engine of
economic growth, the state would offer them only subsistence in the
poorhouses. Charity, justice, and capital accumulation would all
work in sync.

Utilitarianism is a mainstay of public health policy to this day. It
would have been impossible to look at society this way in the plague
era, dominated as it was by church teachings on morality. But the
Enlightenment had opened the window for a new, human-centered
ethical gaze. In particular, the eighteenth-century writing of David
Hume and Adam Smith influenced the developing consciousness
that disease control was obligatory on ethical, not religious, grounds.
Hume wrote in *Enquiry Concerning the Principles of Morals* (1751)
that the human heart "will never be wholly indifferent to public
good." A man might, therefore, make judgments about what others
do even when those deeds don't benefit him directly. Amid the commercial and consumerist atmosphere of that time, disease and the
revealing stench of urban air made it urgent to understand the conditions of life and what cut it short. The new moral gaze made such inquiries virtuous. Epidemics took on moral freight.

Nowhere was the moral valence of epidemic disease more obvious than in America after cholera arrived.

CHOLERA IN AMERICA

Moral indictments of personal habits were already part of the health discussion in America when cholera struck. In New York, where cholera arrived in mid-1832, the Special Medical Council published advice to residents, including abstention from ardent spirits, and issued the reassurance that cholera seemed to affect only the "intemperate and dissolute." The sudden cholera deaths of several prostitutes in Manhattan were taken by some as evidence of the council's point. The higher rates of illness among black and Irish Americans, who were already reputed to be lazy in the first case and drunken in the second, were also seen as evidence. Cholera's preference for immigrant-dense towns and busy ports, where avarice, cunning, and market strategizing had supposedly replaced Christian industriousness, seemed to support the theory.

Thus, while British observers gave the story of epidemic cholera undertones of social change and economic license for industrialists, Americans' text was piety and purity. Like medieval townspeople facing plague, Americans in the 1830s saw cholera as a punishment from God. New York City set aside August 3, 1832, as a day for public fasting and prayer. When the next outbreak began, in 1849, President Zachary Taylor didn't hesitate to establish a national day for humility and prayer, the first Friday in August.

Although some saw cholera as a sign of God's fearsomeness, they were hard-pressed to explain why the Christian God of mercy would send so devastating a scourge to as God-fearing a place as America. A few Protestant clergymen responded to the allegation that cholera was God's weapon in much the way that Clement VII had responded when medieval officials and rabble-rousers attributed plague to the work of Jews: it was sinful temerity to pretend to understand the inscrutable ways of the deity. But Americans generally mixed the spiritual with the plain and the practical: people who were intemperate or indulged in vice brought cholera on themselves.

The attitude in America in the 1830s and '40s was that cholera was a sharp tool for detecting bad behavior. Cholera was supposed to demonstrate that some people, however worshipful they might be, still disobeyed laws of nature: they failed to keep clean, drank too much, indulged in sexual impropriety. People who lived incorrectly in God's world got cholera—including those who were improvident about the practical consequences of their activities and those who violated the standards that were becoming part of the rhetoric of the new Arcadia in America. Harmony with nature was held in high rhetorical esteem (however much it was really strife that characterized Americans' confrontation with their environment); so were temperance with drink, fidelity in marriage, and industriousness at work. As cholera demonstrated, disease in America was to be avoided through proper behavior.

Religious moralists were not the only ones who implicated reprobate behavior as a cause of disease. The founder of the New-York Historical Society wrote in 1832 that cholera was thankfully "almost exclusively confined to the lower classes of intemperate dissolute & filthy people huddled together like swine in their polluted habitations." Not surprisingly, in a country whose self-image was dressed in the conquest of nature and whose social ethos included an abiding belief in the salubriousness of the outdoor life, American medical men saw cholera as a disturbance of the air—an "epidemic influence," some called it, possibly combining with the moral turpitude of impoverished victims. The alleged freshness of American air stood for the health of the collective moral soul of the nation's inhabitants. Ralph Waldo Emerson, writing not long after the first cholera outbreak, was explicit: "I should not be pained at a change which threatened a loss of some of the luxuries or conveniences of society, if it proceeded from a preference of the agricultural life out of the belief, that our primary duties as men could be better discharged in that calling. . . . A man should have a farm or a mechanical craft for his culture."

ILLNESS AND IMMIGRATION

In American hands, the story of an epidemic as a fable illustrating proper behavior inevitably involved national origin. Much was made of the allegation that emigrants from Ireland carried cholera across the Atlantic in 1832, where it entered North America at Montreal. More was made of its subsequent movement southward to New York City in the person of an Irish immigrant named Fitzgerald. The news that the New York outbreak came about not by Irish infiltration but by direct importation via ships sailing in from Europe, known to the city's Board of Health, was quashed in hopes of keeping the outbreak quiet.

Similarly, the 1848–1849 cholera outbreaks in the United States seem to have arisen from numerous near-simultaneous outbreaks in port cities visited by ships from different parts of Europe, although blame was still heaped on the Irish. The German ship *Guttemberg* landed at New Orleans on December 6, 1848, for instance; having sailed out of Hamburg during that city's outbreak, it lost some passengers to cholera during its fifty-five-day journey, then disembarked its roughly 250 surviving steerage passengers in the American city. The *Callao* out of Bremen arrived in New Orleans two days later, also having lost passengers to cholera en route. Cholera then broke out in New Orleans. New York City's outbreak was linked to the arrival of the *New York* out of Le Havre, France, that same month, carrying steerage passengers who, the *New York Times* said, had been forced by bad weather en route to open up baggage—some of which had been packed in Germany, where cholera was raging that autumn. The *Times* pointed out that other ships, from other European ports, had arrived in New York around the same time, and surmised that the city's cholera outbreak resulted when some immigrants escaped from quarantine. The accusation against the Irish simplified the complicated story of the epidemic's spread.

Americans' antipathy toward immigration, which was really antipathy toward immigrants generally (and sometimes, in this largely Protestant country, dislike of Catholics), cloaked itself in cholera fears. Historians of immigration have noted that 1.8 million Irish men, women, and children immigrated to the United States between 1840 and 1860; by the end of that period one-quarter of New York City's residents had been born in Ireland. The *Sunday Times* of New York wrote in 1849, as cholera drew near the city, that "the miserable outcasts are charged with infection on the voyage, and then they are turned loose here to spread ship fever, or whatever contagious disease they may have imbibed." In 1854, another year of cholera outbreaks, the *New York Times* reported on rumors that cholera had broken out among Irish laborers at the suspension bridge at Niagara Falls.

Anger at Irish immigrants for the spread of cholera was voiced loudly through claims about drunkenness. Protestant writers were dismayed about their alleged tolerance for spirits. Charles Rosenberg points out that German immigrants, who were mostly Protestant, were the subjects of less recrimination and fewer allegations of threat—even though they were at least as tolerant of beer drinking as the Irish were of whiskey. Apart from the difference in religion, the Irish were more commonly impoverished, and therefore more often the victims of cholera. In a revealing instance of blaming the victim, the higher cholera mortality among the Irish poor was seen as corroboration that they were carriers of disease. This supposed fact, in turn, corroborated the assumptions about impiety and drink as the real problems.

It was not only because cholera was a disease of the poor, crowded neighborhoods, and therefore the Irish, that it could be shaped into a narrative involving impiety, impurity, and intemperance. Cholera was also useful because it was a disease of cities, especially the mercantile and, by the mid-nineteenth century, rapidly industrializing ports along America's rivers and coastline. Therefore, cholera fit neatly into the American idea that true America was a place of health, fresh air, and toil in the forests or the fields. There were 5,017 deaths in New York City's 1849 outbreak—about 1 percent of the city's population of 515,000. By the time of that outbreak, Americans were complaining that immigrants clustered too much in cities, where they either fomented cholera or suffered from it but in either case were seduced into the urban life of vice. And once tied to the vicious city, immigrants were unable to move out to the land where they might become "real" Americans by helping to clear fields or dig canals. Cholera, along with tuberculosis, typhoid, and smallpox, the other urban contagions of the day, helped to reinforce suspicions of immigration and urban life and furthered the prescriptive nature of American medical thinking: to keep yourself healthy you must lead a pure life of honest labor in the fresh air.

—ɯ—

Cholera disappeared after 1866 as an important outbreak disease in both Europe and the United States, largely as a result of sanitary improvements in cities. Sand filtration of water supplies had begun in London in 1829 and a vast sewer system built by the visionary engineer Joseph Bazalgette opened there in 1865, preventing contamination of drinking water. Philadelphia's Watering Committee was using steam pumps to force fresh water through cast-iron pipes to city residents and industries by 1817. New York had 105 miles of sewer pipes by 1853. Construction of Paris's sewers began under Napoleon, and the sewers were completely separated from the city's water pipes by Baron Haussman's engineers in the 1850s. In the 1860s and '70s, other cities followed the pattern set by London, Paris, and New York, creating separate systems to pipe clean water in and carry waste out. With new urban arrangements in place, cholera outbreaks in Europe and North America decreased in severity after the great one of 1848–1849* and essentially disappeared after the 1890s.

In America, the link between disease and immigration was changing by the time of the last of the large cholera outbreaks. Accusing the poor of bringing their own lot on themselves through filthiness and vice gave way to a spiritually infused social conscience. In the years following the Civil War, the poor were pitied and considered the substrate for reform.

Social reform in America in the second half of the nineteenth century eliminated some of the worst conditions of the life of the poor and developed the urban scene. Importantly, civic improvements afforded the powerful an opportunity to school immigrants in American moral expectations. Big cities were creating standing boards or departments of health empowered to keep streets clean and order quarantine, building sewerage systems and waterworks, and opening hospitals. At the same time, efforts to bring religion to the poor, whose supposed impiety was still deemed a cause of their destitution, increased.

Social thinking about cholera diverged on the two sides of the Atlantic. In America, disease was never far from religious piety, as exemplified in correct behavior. Disease was an aberration of nature, presumed in American ideology to be clement and infused with the spirit of God's working. And medical opinion in America was already attentive to the role of personal habits in creating illness, as it remains today. A Committee on Practical Medicine and Epidemics of the American Medical Association concluded in 1850 that cholera

---

*W. R. E. Smart, in his presidential address to the Epidemiological Society (London) of December 1873, pointed out that there were still some outbreaks (these included Kiev in 1869 and a series of towns in the Mississippi Valley from New Orleans into the upper Midwest in 1873). But they were milder outbreaks.

was known to be caused by individuals' impropriety or intemperance. Ideas about cholera were subsumed in broader notions about what was good in America. In Europe, cholera was the stage for political maneuvering around miasmas and became a weapon in the arsenal of liberal capitalism, bent on fixing the problems of poverty by coercing the poor into the labor force. On both sides of the ocean, cholera heralded the opening of campaigns that made use of epidemic disease for political ends.

—ᴠᴠ—

I love the forest. It is bad to live in cities: there,
too many are in heat.

—Friedrich Nietzsche,
Thus Spoke Zarathustra

Maybe all of the thinking about epidemic disease in the first three-quarters of the nineteenth century was no more than a way of attributing illness and the poverty that was assumed to result from it to the people who suffered from them most: the laboring classes who clustered by necessity in industrial cities, living in squalor. It would have been hard to put such accusations into words by talking simply about cholera, typhus, diphtheria, typhoid, or TB, the common communicable killers of the indigent. The obvious truth that the urban poor were so sick would have been merely descriptive; it would not have ascribed to the indigent a role in their own tribulations. To educated middle-class Englishmen, pious Americans, apologists for industrialization and its reshaping of the landscape, or believers in the Emersonian vision of American outdoor work or the Jeffersonian vision of an agrarian democracy—really, to any of the people of the 1800s for whom hordes of the destitute living in squalor was inexplicable or just offensive—the framing of the epidemic around bad air, bad water, or bad habits neatly explained the way that disease concentrated where the poor did. It also implied that cholera and its dire companions weren't really anyone's fault, just the cost of doing business.

The advent of germ theory not long after cholera outbreaks subsided would change epidemic thought, but the residue of miasma-era thinking remains in today's assumptions about epidemics. The old struggles over smells, air, and illness are evident in inquiries into the particular effects of place on disease occurrence. Nobody can explain how *E. coli* 0157:H7 got into spinach that was ultimately sold at market and sickened many people in 2006, but we understand it had something to do with the ecosystem in California's Central Valley. We think of the poor neighborhoods of modern-day cities (if we think of them at all) as breeding grounds for illness—we're aware of the high rates of asthma, diabetes, and AIDS. We can't explain this in terms of germs or any specific cause. We no longer say that the air in some neighborhoods is bad for people's health, but it seems that way. Miasma failed at specifying what actually causes disease in individuals, but the idea had a certain strength to it: no one thing makes the health of the poor worse. It's a kind of environmental stress, and it has to do with the conjunction of place and disease.

CHAPTER 4

GERMS, SCIENCE,
AND THE STRANGER

It makes me furious, such things beholding:
From Water, Earth, and Air unfolding,
A thousand germs break forth and grow.

—JOHANN WOLFGANG VON GOETHE,
MEPHISTOPHELES

In *Faust*, when Goethe's Mephistopheles refers to "a thousand germs" (*tausend Keime*) he means embryos, seeds, spores—"germ" as the principle of life. And yet the line sounds to the modern ear like a description of the fearsome swarm unleashed—one that recalls a burst of cases of the severe acute respiratory syndrome (SARS), which debuted in Hong Kong in 2003, or reports of methicillin-resistant *Staphylococcus aureus* (MRSA), responsible, in the words of federal officials, for "more U.S. deaths than AIDS."

SARS burst into the news in February 2003, after more than three hundred cases of an unusual pneumonia were reported to the World Health Organization (WHO) from China, with five deaths. The outbreak had begun in November of the previous year in farm communities in Guangdong Province, in southern China. It spread quickly, carried by travelers. In mid-March, with cases having been reported from Hanoi (in a man who had traveled from Hong Kong), Singapore, and Canada, the WHO issued global health alerts. By August 2003, 5,327 cases and 349 deaths had been reported in China. Worldwide, there were 8,098 cases and 774 deaths.

SARS, the "first epidemic of the twenty-first century," as some put it, was noisy but swift. The first cases appeared in mid-November 2002; the last cases in July 2003. By late summer it was over. But SARS resonated in an atmosphere already alert to "emerging infections" and "bioterrorism." The *New York Times* ran more than two hundred articles on SARS in 2003; *The Globe and Mail* published more than three hundred. The public television network PBS ran two or three stories each month.

The resonance extended to, and was perhaps amplified by, documented cases of SARS transmission on commercial air flights. Unlike tuberculosis, which does not spread easily through cabin air, the SARS-associated virus does seem to be transmissible from a sick person to passengers seated nearby. During the 2003 outbreak, the virus, a member of the coronavirus family called SARS-coV, seems to have been passed from person to person during a few flights, ones that were more than ninety minutes long. Recognizing what looked like a global threat, several airports in Asia and Canada instituted thermal-scanning procedures to detect travelers who had fever: 35.7 million passengers were screened, but only 4,177 (about one out of every 10,000 screenings) turned out to have fever. And not one case of SARS was detected.

Intense outbreaks of SARS occurred in three medical centers in the Toronto area, where nearly a hundred health-care workers were infected. Officials asked 3,000 people in the Toronto area who had been exposed to SARS to go into isolation for ten days, to avoid infecting others. The Toronto-area SARS outbreak prompted the WHO to issue an advisory in April 2003 warning travelers that Toronto was a spot best avoided for the time being.

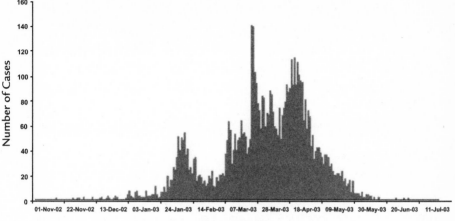

The epidemic of severe acute respiratory syndrome (SARS). This figure shows the pattern of new diagnoses for 5,910 cases worldwide from November 2002 through mid-July 2003 (2,527 reported cases are not included in this graph because dates of onset were unknown). *Source:* World Health Organization, *Consensus Document on the Severe Acute Respiratory Syndrome (SARS)*, 2003, available at http://www.who.int/csr/sars/en/WHOconsensus.pdf (downloaded December 6, 2008), 8.

With airplanes involved; travel advisories reminiscent of blizzards, hurricanes, or floods; and the clamor about global catastrophe imparting to SARS a contemporary cachet, the keynotes of modernity started to sound. By mid-March 2003, SARS was being called the "jet-borne killer disease" and "the first jet-set plague." Its agent was known simply as the "super-bug." By early April, "SARS" was the second most common search term in Google, a rumor was spreading online that SARS was the result of genetic experiments gone awry, and an e-mail discussion group on SARS took the title "The New Plague." Plans for bioterrorism response were readied. The Rolling Stones canceled two concerts in Hong Kong. Morgan Stanley lowered its economic forecast for Asia.

Investigators on the trail of the SARS agent identified so-called superspreaders.* A person known as Patient ZH in Guangzhou, China, was held responsible for eighty-two cases in which people were infected by "aerosolizing incidents" (another jet-age term) in two hospitals where ZH had been interned. A large cluster of cases occurred at the Amoy Gardens apartment complex in Hong Kong. Sixteen cases were reported at the Metropole Hotel in Kowloon. The Metropole cluster later gave rise to further outbreaks in Toronto, Hanoi, and Singapore when former guests of the hotel traveled to those cities. Five "superspreaders" in Singapore accounted for more than one hundred additional cases.

There was much hype about the twenty-first-century plague, yet the SARS outbreak was contained by very old-fashioned techniques: keeping the sick away from the well and the possibly infected away from the definitely uninfected. Quarantines were used, and voluntary isolation, travel advisories, doctors' and nurses' masks—not so different from the precautions of the days of the Black Death. Indeed, there were scenes that might have come from the fourteenth century: universities in Beijing were shut down, three hundred students of one university were sent to a quarantine camp outside the city, and entire dormitories in other universities were quarantined. Schools were closed for two weeks, and 1.7 million Beijing children were kept home. Two thousand patients and health workers were shut inside Beijing University People's Hospital facility. Another 2,000 were ordered into quarantine. Thousands

---

*It does seem that some people with SARS-coV are more infectious than others (that is, more likely to transmit a microorganism to contacts). This is true for many forms of contagion. Probably, high infectivity arises out of a conjunction of circumstances, involving particular interactions between the virus or bacterium in question and the genetically determined internal chemical environment of the sick person, transient aspects of the immune state of the individual, and the specifics of how that person interacts with others.

fled Beijing, but hotels outside the city closed to travelers who had been in the capital. Within Beijing, movie theaters and dance halls shut. "People and cars not from this village are forbidden to enter," read a sign outside a town near Beijing. Outside another Chinese town, a reporter found vigilantes standing with bottles of disinfectant, ready to spray anyone who entered. In another, villagers attacked and tried to burn a center that the government had designated as a SARS quarantine facility. Some Chinese banks sterilized banknotes. In Taiwan, taxi drivers refused to pick up people outside the gates of Shanxi Province People's Hospital. The government in Taiwan suspended travel permits for people coming from Guangzhou and Shanxi provinces, Inner Mongolia, and Beijing. In Malaysia, 284 patients and staff in a mental hospital were shut into quarantine.

Yet amid the panic, containment procedures worked as they often had in the past. Of the 774 SARS fatalities worldwide, almost all were in China, including Hong Kong and Taiwan: outside, there were thirty-three deaths in Singapore and forty-three in Canada—and even there, the outbreaks were touched off by travelers returning after the Metropole Hotel event in Hong Kong. There were only sporadic fatalities elsewhere: five in Vietnam, two in the Philippines, one each in a number of countries. For all its supposed talent for airplane travel, the SARS virus managed to move only briefly, sparking outbreaks that were explosive enough to elude control measures and produce substantial mortality only in the Toronto area and Singapore. The force of the SARS wave was otherwise feeble and relatively easy to contain.

About 8,000 people made ill and nearly 800 deaths made for a grievous event. But SARS was not a world catastrophe, not even tantamount to a moderately severe year of influenza or one month's worth of traffic accidents in the United States. SARS turned out to be amenable to control. It was transmitted only by sick people, primarily by droplets of sputum or saliva (which can't travel too far).

Once it was clear that sick people had to be isolated and that their caregivers had to take precautions to prevent infection, the chains of transmission were broken.

SARS obeyed the classic plague paradigm, but on a limited scale. Maybe that's why it was easy to speak of it as "the first epidemic of the twenty-first century." First there was nothing, then a report of a severe outbreak. A few cases were revealed, then suddenly there were very many, then few . . . then none. From the initial report in early February 2003, the numbers of new cases rose through mid-April. Then, with the intensity of new outbreaks at its greatest, it was only eleven weeks until SARS was completely gone.

GERM THEORY VICTORIOUS

The triumph of germ theory explains both why we can control diseases like SARS and why we are terrified by them. Germ theory allows us to see human illness as the result of a pathogenic process begun by infection with a single microorganism. There should be a different illness for each microbe: *Yersinia pestis* makes plague, *Vibrio cholerae* causes cholera, *Mycobacterium tuberculosis* TB, *Bacillus anthracis* anthrax, and so forth. The spread of any illness is the human manifestation of the movements of the respective germ.

The simplicity of the one-bug-causes-one-disease view was well suited to the mood of twentieth-century modernity. The growth of the middle classes; sharper distinctions between the middle and laboring classes; the middle classes' willingness to adhere to mores of cleanliness and sexual propriety; the shifting of moral reproof from religious impiety to behavioral impropriety; industrialized economies' need to sell manufactured products; manufacturers' desire to highlight health threats that could be fended off with their products; and a penchant for seeing struggle not as a constant fact of life but as an opportunity to demonstrate the validity of a grand ideology—all of these hallmarks of modern industrial society were served by the notion that an epidemic has a single cause. To think that disease out-breaks result when a microbe exploits the faulty activity of a single cog in the social machine—one individual, that is—is to hold to a belief that one mistake can sicken the whole population.

In earlier times, people had blamed the unwanted; it was the very identity of the dispossessed that implicated them as spreaders of whatever plague was current: lepers, the Jews, foreigners, impover-ished Irishmen. But in a world where money and power are guided not by land ownership and allegiances to home village but by indus-trial productivity, birthright matters less than behavior.

The simple causal story in which germs had been allowed to in-filtrate society because a few individuals behaved ineptly or incon-siderately remains compelling. In the 1980s, it allowed for accounts of AIDS to begin with the "greatest [gay] party ever known," in the words of one author, or, in another's telling, with the "anonymous sexuality" of "multiple-partnering on an unprecedented scale." The simple causal story is why, in the United States in the early 1990s, expanding urban poverty created by years of Reagonomics, the crack-cocaine wars, incarceration policies, and AIDS combined to stall the decline in rates of TB (incidence actually increased for a while), yet so-called resurgent tuberculosis was attributed to the fail-ure of TB patients to take their antibiotic medication. It is why syphilis was blamed on prostitutes and "loose women" a hundred years ago and why, even now, upturns in syphilis rates are blamed on gay men who have "relapsed" into "unsafe sex." In a way, germ theory was perfect for an era of productivity. It knit the disapproval of nonstandard behavior with anxieties about new technology. The epidemic became a matter of people doing the wrong thing (and do-ing it with the wrong people), a matter of too much freedom to mix and make mischief.

That the way people understand an epidemic was infiltrated by germs and germ theory so thoroughly, quickly, and durably is testa-ment to the real, messy, complicated (and money-driven) nature of scientific revolutions and to the power in modern society of scientific change to revise the public conversation.

—⟋𝖂⟍—

Now that we know so much about viruses and bacteria and the illnesses they help cause, it is tempting to view the rise of germ theory as a steady progression of information accumulation and rational inference. We might read the history of the amassing of evidence in favor of germ theory in the 1870s, '80s, and '90s—the laboratory cultures, histological stains, "passaging" of tissue from one animal to another, the isolation of the germ—as a matter of the gradual acquisition of supportive evidence. We might think that strong evidence in favor of germ theory simply overwhelmed incredulity, so that rational thinkers were forced by scientific logic to abandon other theories. Indeed, much modern writing on the topic makes germ theory seem so well supported by accumulating evidence that rational people who were concerned with health examined it and found it believable, persuasive, and, finally, incontrovertible.

But the winning scientific theory isn't always the only correct one. Germ theory was propelled forward by a kind of force of arms in the form of rapidly developing tools for laboratory science. In a world increasingly attentive to science as a source of truth, microbiologists' capacity to provide evidence from the laboratory that would back their assertions gave them the edge in the struggle to be heard. Without the laboratory, germ theory could not have cleared away competing contenders to come to dominate thinking about epidemics.

How germ theory became the sole truth of contagion is a social story, not just a matter of scientists evaluating evidence. No theory about disease's spread at any time has been accepted so universally as the germ model in the modern era. Germ theory won supremacy as an explanation for disease by overcoming miasmatism, anti-contagionism, religious explanations, astrological beliefs, the vitalism of homeopaths, and yet more concepts. By the 1890s, the single, clear voice of germ theory muted all other accounts of why outbreaks happen.

Importantly for the rise of germ theory, a central force in Western society in the nineteenth century was industry's ability to overcome natural obstacles in the pursuit of productivity. New problem-solving techniques, the increasing prosperity of many in industrializing countries, and the concomitantly widening gap between the destitute and the rest of society also helped to position germ theory as the answer everyone was waiting for. The illumination of the mysteries of nature also played a part.

—⚮—

Mysteries had been the coin of religion in medieval times, but by the 1800s the tale in which nature's secrets are unveiled through human effort and intellect had become popular. Poe introduced the detective novel with *Murders in the Rue Morgue* in 1841; within a generation, Wilkie Collins had published his mystery novels *The Woman in White* (1859) and *The Moonstone* (1868); Sherlock Holmes entered the world in 1881 in *A Study in Scarlet* (and kept going through Conan Doyle's last story in 1927, then reappeared in film, books, comics, and television). The detective triumphs over nature, revealing the mystery to be a matter of intelligible mechanics: the murderer of the Baskerville men was no uncanny hound from hell; it was (Holmes sagely concludes) a human seeking fortune and status. Those aspects of nature that remained unknowable and invisible, unavailable to human decoding, were the more horrifying—as the popularity of vampire yarns in the nineteenth century attests.

In a sense, nineteenth-century society was *looking* for germs. People were searching not merely for explanations of disease outbreaks like cholera but for a vision of what might be beyond the visible world. They wanted experts to seek out clues, but they remained wary of the uncanny that undermined the security of modern life.

The security of modern life was an open question by the middle of the nineteenth century. Policy makers turned their attention to social conditions, and the new middle classes made demands for government liberalization. Unrest spread around Europe in 1848: the February Revolution in France inaugurated the Second Republic and called for right-to-work laws; the March Revolutions in the German-speaking states included demands for civil rights. The rise of communism and other labor movements directed attention to the conditions of workers and their families. The Second Empire rose and fell in France, and war was waged between France and Prussia in 1870–1871. Amid the social and political turmoil at midcentury, the way people understood an epidemic changed. The epidemic story had to accommodate fears of death, disability, social instability, and the random, mortal bite of nature.

By midcentury, the very nature of illness had all the resonance of a complicated social phenomenon. Understanding disease outbreaks meant recognizing the impact of social and economic life. An epidemic prevented crops from being harvested, kept men out of work, and killed people when the rains failed to fall or crops failed to grow.

Epidemiology, the study of epidemic illness, was more than just scaffolding for describing disease outbreaks. In 1830, a French surgeon-turned-social economist, Louis-René Villermé, published the seminal article on epidemiology when he reported his research on the differential mortality in Parisian *arrondissements*. Villermé had explored many plausible factors in search of an explanation for the variation of death rates from one neighborhood of the city to another, including elevation, proximity to the Seine, population density, and extent of open space. The one determinant that lined up closely with mortality rate was the proportion of the population that was too poor to pay taxes: the poorest neighborhoods had the highest mortality and the wealthiest the lowest. In fact, wealthy French people lived about one and a half times longer than their poorest compatriots at the time. For Villermé and his fellows in the *partie d'hygiene*, the Hygiene Group, poverty was the impediment, blocking access to the individual liberty that the French Revolution had promised. Villermé was among the first researchers to use statistics to demonstrate how disease is entangled with social life.

The pathologist Rudolf Virchow saw the same connection between social deprivation and illness. In 1848, he was sent to Upper Silesia by Prussia's minister of education to examine conditions among the peasants. Typhus had broken out and had literally decimated the destitute.

Typhus is a louse-borne illness, resulting from infection with the tiny bacterium *Rickettsia prowazekii*. The body louse, *Pediculus humanus*, is an inhabitant of body hair and clothing; lice are ubiquitous among people living in crowded conditions who are unable to wash themselves or their clothes. The louse ingests bacteria when it bites an infected person. If that same louse bites another person within a few days of taking in the bacteria, it excretes some of them in its feces. When the person rubs or scratches the louse bite (or, sometimes, when lice are crushed against the skin), the excreted *Rickettsia* are driven into and through the skin, whence they can enter the bloodstream. A louse thus infected is capable of spreading the illness to other people nearby. Not surprisingly, typhus is a well-known companion of people suffering famine or displaced by war; malnourishment contributes to the pathogenesis.

After extensive study of the typhus outbreak in Upper Silesia, Virchow concluded that contagion could not be alleviated by medical treatment alone; it required, he wrote, "radical action to promote the advancement of an entire population." In order to prevent the spread of illness, Virchow insisted, education, liberty, and prosperity must be guaranteed. Palliative approaches to disease would no longer work. Only the "radical action" of social remediation would improve standards of living, Virchow asserted, and only improved living standards would both uplift the poor morally and protect the population from outbreaks of contagion.

Epidemiology became a tool with which to address the effect of social problems on disease and quell fears of the haphazard. With its statistics and wide scope, the study of epidemics grew swiftly in prominence, keenly attuned to social conditions.

The first association of men interested in studying epidemics, the London Epidemiological Society, was founded in March 1850. Headed by Dr. Benjamin Babington of Guy's Hospital, the LES's first meeting was attended by a hundred English physicians and others alert to the need to apply science to prevent further disasters like the cholera outbreak of 1848–1849.

The Society was bound to examine epidemics as a threat to the civil state. From the outset, its aims were not only to carry out scientific studies of causes and conditions that influence the occurrence and spread of disease but also to communicate with government bodies the results of new research into the "laws of disease," so as to help prevent epidemics. "So far as we are able," Babington declaimed in his inaugural address, "having made ourselves thoroughly acquainted with the strongholds of our enemies, and their modes of attack, [our object is] . . . to seek how they may be most effectually combated and expelled."

THE BIRTH AND GROWTH OF EPIDEMIOLOGY

Epidemiology effectively tied social life to medicine and helped bring a scientific cachet to the medical arts, expanding the physician's view outward from his consulting office to the city and the nation. But there was no how-to manual for epidemiology in 1850. Statistics became its main tool, evolving as a set of methods tied very much to the conception of the epidemic as a deadly invasion—because death is one of the easy-to-identify and broadly meaningful events by which health and disease can be measured. Medical statistics had already been recognized as a field of study by the early 1800s (Gottfried Achenwall first used the word Statistik, from the Latin *status*, meaning "state," in 1748, to designate methods by which a government analyzes the strength of a state by collecting and studying numerical information on birth, disease, and death). William Farr, registrar general of England, wanted health statistics to pave the route to social reform, focusing particularly on the use of life tables to study probabilities of dying. Epidemiology was thus based on mortality risk: the proportion of fatalities, the probability statement as to how likely it is that members of one population will die and the comparison of that group's chances with another's.

Risk resonates with the human sense of peril, hazard, and dire consequence. Risk also denotes a statistical prediction of what is likely to happen to an individual, a method that was already in use by the nineteenth century for the purposes of setting insurance premiums. The statements that epidemiologists made about the probability of illness or death in a large population eventually came to be uttered in the language of risk. That has made them sound like warnings about danger to individuals, however much epidemiologists strive to talk only about populations. In other words, from its beginnings, risk allied the study of epidemics to both collective dread and individual chances. With risk carrying different but related meanings, epidemiology came to occupy a curious position—fraught with the culture's sense of peril in the form of illness, attentive to the life chances of individuals, but looking broadly at the conditions of society.

Soon after its founding, the London Epidemiological Society formed committees on smallpox, cholera, fevers, and hospitals, and was particularly interested in supplying nurses for the poor. Although its members debated the mechanisms by which diseases spread, epidemiologists at the middle of the nineteenth century managed to know how to prevent the spread of disease without any exclusive theory of contagion. Smallpox, they knew, could be prevented by vaccination, and a sufficiently heavily vaccinated population would resist smallpox outbreaks. Typhus could be controlled if the people did not want for food and shelter. Cleaning the cities and, especially, providing pure water and constructing sewerage systems suppressed cholera outbreaks.

Early epidemiologists were undecided about germs, though. Virchow himself refused to accept the idea of germ causation of disease, preferring the view that illness was an outgrowth of complex causes, social as well as biological. When Friedrich Gustav Jakob Henle, known as the Father of Germ Theory, postulated in 1840 that contagious diseases were spread by living microscopic organisms, he was summarizing more than a century and a half of thinking on the topic, trying to organize and clarify the confusing and sometimes contradictory ideas about the spread of disease. But Henle's microorganism approach met with considerable opposition as a theory of disease. A germ theory would tend to undermine the physicians' craft, since doctors' work was based on knowledge of the patient and attention to observable signs, not microscopic creatures. And in a time of industrialization, political ferment, and social change, respectable epidemiologists in London and hygienists in Paris would not embrace a theory that discounted the role of social circumstances in disease formation.

Opposition to germ theory arose on political grounds, as well. By the early nineteenth century, the possibility of contagion had become a useful rationale for demanding that foreign ships undergo sanitary inspections and using quarantine as a way of regulating trade. By midcentury, though, a nation's interest might seem better served by opening markets so its industrialists could move their products. Quarantines that would help protect home businesses also impeded commercial expansion. An anti-quarantine movement took shape, fueled by economics and adopting a mishmash of ideas about disease that collectively came to be called "anti-contagionism." Some held to a telluric theory, in which disease was caused by some sort of seismic emanations, while others espoused an electrical theory involving ozone. The movement seems to have existed primarily to debunk the inconvenient notion that interdicting invisible germs or seeds through slowing trade or limiting industry could also prevent illness.

Anti-contagionist arguments were shepherded by pro-trade forces and their political allies, the liberals. Some liberal reformers were likely attracted to anti-contagionism because they disapproved of the deprivation of liberty that quarantine required. Others joined in because they could not abide the notion, implicit in quarantine, that everyone is equally vulnerable to disease—universal suscepti-bility erases distinctions between the educated middle and upper classes, on the one hand, and the poor, on the other. In the view of English liberals and American reformers, the epidemic was defined by the educated and driven by impropriety.

The anti-contagionist cause benefited from a commonly held bias that illness had more to do with inherent predispositions than external causes. Physicians in England complied with this notion, asserting that cholera was a type of fever that tended to affect those who were most readily disposed to it because of poverty or immoral habits. In the United States, idleness and drink were the cause of poverty and the "parent of disease," as a publication of the 1830s put it. Some people held that the popular miasma theory meant that ill-nesses like cholera were not really contagious, explaining the occur-rence of different diseases on the basis of the interaction of vapors on the differing constitutional predispositions of the people exposed to the noxious air. Predisposition was paramount.

—ɯ—

The rise of epidemiology as an extension of the physician's practice and the debate about contagion and predisposition were part of the expanding role of doctors in the nineteenth century, especially in the United States and Britain. Doctors plied their trade with vigor, seeking leverage to edge out competition from other medicine-related professions (surgeons, on the one hand; herbalists and homeopaths, on the other): publicity, especially in the form of medical and scien-tific journals, played an important role in professionalizing physician-hood. So did professional organizations such as the American Medical

Association and the Royal Society of Medicine, the new guilds. Lob-
bying to influence legislation was another sign of professionalization.
But one of the most important ways for physicians to demonstrate to
the public that their profession was both legitimate and forward-
looking was to embrace laboratory science.

By the last quarter of the nineteenth century, new technologies
promoting success in industry had shown their usefulness in building
economic power, and new weaponry had changed the outcome of
wars (including, prominently, Gatling's machine gun in the American Civil War and Krupp's breech-loaded six-pound cannon in the
Austro-Prussian and Franco-Prussian wars). The laboratory would
show its own capacity to expand economic and political power by
turning technical know-how into useful knowledge.

Thus the milieu for technical advance in the name of science
was favorable at the end of the 1800s. Expanding economies in the
industrializing countries meant more opportunity for scientific research. With a growing bourgeoisie, more people had an education
and the time and inclination for learning through study and experimentation. And with new economic classes having the leisure for
higher education, both universities and laboratories expanded. The
circumstances of life—the impact of society, environment, and education on behavior—were scrutinized.

MICROBIOLOGY'S DEBUT

A signal event in the rise of germ theory was the isolation of the
causal agent of anthrax in 1876 by a former student of Henle's,
Robert Koch. Capitalizing on the favorable attitude toward science,
Koch developed techniques in microbiology, contributing to the
study of microorganisms and the identification of numerous other
important pathogens: with his methods the causative agents of
syphilis, gonorrhea, typhoid, pneumonia, meningitis, plague, and
tetanus were discovered. In 1882, Koch identified the tuberculosis

bacillus. A year later, he identified the cholera vibrio.* In France, Louis Pasteur was advancing the study of the mechanisms of microbial infection and methods for modifying susceptibility.

By the end of the 1890s, Koch's innovations in laboratory technique and Pasteur's insights into infection, along with the observations and laboratory work of many of their followers, had led to the identification of agents associated with about a dozen and a half human and animal diseases. These included the different bacteria responsible for typhoid, leprosy, tuberculosis, cholera, gangrene, botulism, dysentery, and plague, as well as the streptococcus and staphylococcus. By 1910, physician scientists had established that individuals who were infected with an organism could infect others, even if they seemed unaffected by the illness it caused—these so-called carriers either having already recovered from the ailment in question or never having shown any symptoms in the first place. Combining observation with laboratory studies, medical scientists had shown that carriers were responsible for the spread of cholera, diphtheria, and typhoid fever within communities. Soon thereafter, the general importance of carriers became clear, and the carrier came to figure as an important element of the modern conception of the epidemic—a convenient substitute for the bedeviled.

Evidence for germ theory took on added authority because it came from experiments in the laboratory, the new temple of technology. Had there been less support for laboratory work (support that came from both government and private industry), less tendency to credit laboratory science, or less dogged persistence on the part of the proponents of microbiology like Koch and Pasteur, germ theory might not have posted so impressive a record of discovery, and would have been less able to assure itself of attention by a world ready to take on the problem of illness.

---

*The vibrio had been isolated previously, in 1854, by Filippo Pacini, but his discovery was largely ignored at the time.

EVOLUTION, SOCIAL DARWINISM,
AND THE CARRIER

The triumph of germ theory had to do not only with the evolution of technology and revolutions both industrial and social; it also had to do with the revolution in thinking about the natural world that Charles Darwin set off.

Darwin's seminal work, *On the Origin of Species by Means of Natural Selection,* appeared in November 1859. The doctrine of natural selection turned Carl Linnaeus's eighteenth-century taxonomy of the plant and animal kingdoms (phyla, orders, classes, and so forth) into a hierarchy—and, although this wasn't Darwin's explicit intent, placed humankind at the top. Natural selection made differences seem inherent to the nature of humans and seemed to signal that all creatures interacted with the world through varying degrees of struggle. Looked at through the evolutionary lens, humanity's clash with potentially life-threatening diseases held a significance much beyond an individual's desire to survive. Surviving illness mattered to the species, to humankind.

If natural selection seemed to imply a duty to the species, so-called social Darwinism reframed the understanding of epidemics. Herbert Spencer coined the term "survival of the fittest" in his 1864 book, *Principles of Biology.* Both Spencer and German zoologist Ernst Haeckel proposed that the same natural evolutionary processes Darwin described in the wild govern the relation of individual humans to society: social evolution tends toward the perfection of humankind. In Spencer's view, those who better adapt to circumstance do better socially (and therefore economically)—a claim that became the rationale for a moral interpretation of evolutionary science. Haeckel went further, asserting that an artificial selection must be imposed atop natural selection, preventing social misfits such as criminals from transmitting their hereditary criminality to the next generation. As the British physiologist John Haycraft proposed, infectious diseases could exert a natural selection "friend[ly] to the race," culling the unfit. Preventing infection among the worthy could provide artificial selection—helping the higher orders survive assaults by lower orders of nature (that is, by germs). The old dread of social instability reappeared in Darwinian clothes.

Germ theory also offered social Darwinists a chance to advance an explanation for society's economic realities. In answering why certain groups of people seemed to remain destitute, social Darwinists pointed to hereditary susceptibilities. Such people, in the social Darwinists' view, weren't as fit or immune and couldn't escape infection. When they got sick, they couldn't work. Ergo, they remained poor.

Germ theory let the social Darwinists tag the less deserving with a logic that was flawed but nonetheless resonant with sound science: if you believed that disease rates differed from one group to another because of some intrinsic, biological, and therefore natural social ordering, then you could conclude that the poor were kept destitute by their tendency to get sick. As higher disease rates *were* observed among certain peoples, such as the Irish in England and the United States, Africans and their descendants in America, and soon in other immigrant groups to the United States who came to be defined as separate races, like Jews and Italians, the inference that those people were less fit seemed validated. Their tendency to get sick could be dismissed as a consequence of natural forces, a lower evolutionary status. The lower orders of humans, the social Darwinist could claim, were less removed in the evolutionary scheme from the microbes that cause the illness than were the more advanced types.

To turn disease clustering into a sign of diminished fitness required a misreading of both evolution and epidemiology. We do this today, although more subtly. It is what is implied when our news programs about AIDS, filariasis, or tuberculosis in Africa include many shots of troupes of dark-skinned people in native costume performing tribal dances and, equally, lethargic toddlers with swollen stomachs, but not a single scene of people in Western clothes, driving to work, using computers, or playing with their kids in suburban yards—as if Africans were mired in the nineteenth century. It is what we mean when we say that there are grave and worrying disparities in cancer survival between white Americans and African Americans, and when we go on to correlate African American "ethnicity" with susceptibility to prostate cancer, as a recent scientific report does. It is what we mean when we claim, as a recent article in a peer-reviewed epidemiology journal does, that race is associated with higher levels of "risk behavior" (in this case, smoking cigarettes and marijuana and drinking alcohol). We reify race whenever we associate it with presumptively noxious, morally reproved behaviors. When we imagine that a group has some extra susceptibility to a particular germ, as many people did when AIDS turned out to strike black Americans at higher rates than white Americans, we continue the social Darwinist misuse of germ theory to solidify race-based causal thinking, equating infection with biological defect.

The logic of germs and genes helps make race seem like a biological thing. If you believed this form of reasoning in the nineteenth century, then cholera among the Irish in the United States and Britain, yellow fever among African Americans, and, by the 1890s, tuberculosis among Jewish emigrants from Russia were simply signs of lower evolutionary status. Never mind that the Irish in the 1840s and '50s were too poor to live in sanitary parts of the cities where they labored; never mind that black men were employed on docks in swampy or riverside zones where mosquitoes were constantly present; never mind that the Russian Jews crowded into airless tenements on the Lower East Side of New York: epidemic disease simply demonstrated the logic of evolution. Race has long been a useful concept for people who have sought to allay their distress about the haphazard and unpredictable threat of deadly illness.

Germ theory offered a neat marker by which suspect groups could be identified as races—it provided a rationale for prejudice, with scientific backing and the guise of disease control to mask what is really discrimination. When the old certainty that an epidemic is a complex social phenomenon gave way to the new belief that an epidemic is a simple matter of infection with germs, suspicions about genetic predisposition and hereditary fitness moved to the forefront of thinking about public health. No need to redistribute resources or keep the water clean for everyone. Some people can't be helped.

GERMS IN AMERICA

In the United States, germ theory did not catch on as quickly as it did in Europe, consumed as American physicians were with the matter of predisposition. But germs provided a way to talk about the ineffable American worries, about race preeminently but also about national origin and class. And once germ theory aligned with the characteristically American concerns about probity and piety, it was an American hit.

Even after the bacteriological revolution of the 1880s, American physicians preferred to see disease in the framework of "seed and soil": heredity and environment combine to produce illness—together they constitute the fertile "soil" that allows an accidental "seeding" by germs to become pathological. It was predisposition that determined where microbes might successfully seed and therefore really decided whether an infection would generate illness. The seed-and-soil metaphor meant that, as a paper read at the 1884 American Public Health Association meeting put it, "a predisposition, i.e., a congenial soil is necessary for the development and growth of the specific . . . germ."

In the seed-and-soil view, disease outbreaks inevitably accompanied life in the industrialized city and were intimately associated with improper behavior. In the late nineteenth century, tuberculosis, the leading cause of death and thus the leading example, was thought to have a preference for the factory worker, the poor, and the dark-skinned. A medical textbook of 1881 was explicit on this matter: TB is caused by heredity and climate, it said, along with a sedentary life, lack of fresh outdoor air and sunlight, and depressive mood. Robert Koch's claim, in 1882, that the TB bacillus was the constant cause of all forms of TB disease was greeted with skepticism in the United States; a respected pathologist at the University of Pennsylvania described Koch's theory as "far too one-sided to have an application to scientific medicine." The view that what matters most in disease occurrence is the innate susceptibility of the potential victim was already so ingrained that the president of the American Public Health Association objected to Koch's claim that a specific germ could invariably cause TB: he warned that "associated influences," like "misery, loss of sleep, [and] malnutrition," would be overlooked if germ theory got too much credence.

It might seem that the American version of germ theory, with its emphasis on predisposition, opened the door to the kind of social reform the epidemiologists of the 1840s and '50s—Virchow, Farr, and others—saw as essential to the control of disease. But the American agenda was much more focused on personal habits—and the supposed perniciousness of particular, unpopular styles of living.

"Seed and soil" served the physicians' purpose. Even as more evidence was amassed on the role of germs in the transmission of disease, American health advocates continued to attribute disease to reprobate behaviors and city life. A leading result was the tuberculosis sanatorium.* Sanatoriums were meant to get disease sufferers out of the supposedly noxious urban environment and cultivate

---

*Sanatoriums had existed before the bacteriologic era—to house the incurable, for instance, or (in imitation of German rest spas, the *Kurorten*) to offer pleasant surroundings and country air. Examples were the Cragmoor in Colorado Springs and Mountain Sanitorium [sic] in Asheville, North Carolina. Adirondack Cottage, founded at Saranac Lake, New York, in 1885, picked up the spa idea and changed it. Its founder, E. L. Trudeau, having recovered from TB himself, said in his 1903 essay "The History of the Tuberculosis Work at Saranac Lake, New York" (*Medical News* 83, no. 2) that he believed that "it is not so much where the consumptive lives as *how* he lives that is important" [emphasis added]. Followers of Adirondack Cottage included White Haven in Pennsylvania, Loomis in Liberty, New York, and Barlow in Los Angeles.

"healthy" habits of eating, sleeping, bathing, and exercising, along with abstention from alcohol, so as to build resistance. In the process, the tubercular patient was removed from society. As with the insane, for whom sanatoriums had been the standard place of internment, the tubercular person went into exile in the sanatorium.

Other expressions of the epidemic imagination in late-nineteenth-century America were more invidious than the sanatorium. The nativist movement put germs to its own use, making the prevention of contagion a rationale for excluding immigrants. Nativists clamored for exclusion of Chinese based on assumptions that Chinese people harbored tuberculosis, syphilis, and other contagious illnesses. They accused Italian immigrants of spreading polio and contributing to the degradation of the white race (of which Italians were not considered a part) by polluting the gene pool. They claimed that Jews immigrating from the Russian Pale of Settlement brought tuberculosis.

Nativists' specific allegations about immigrants reveal just how far germs and genes had penetrated the political consciousness— and how they might serve the ends of the powerful. Since germs couldn't be seen and sometimes gave no sign of their presence yet were supposed to be contagious, the fearful easily turned accusatory, suspecting that presumed germ carriers were treacherous degraders of respectable society.

In 1870, after the physician Arthur Stout had published a tract on "Chinese Immigration and the Physiological Causes of the Decay of a Nation" in which he alleged that Chinese people harbored numerous dangerous illnesses, the California Board of Health hired him to study how Chinese "hereditary vices and engrafted peculiarities" posed a threat to their state's population through racial admixture. By 1876 Californians were claiming that the Chinese would spread leprosy in the United States and, by exposing Americans to disease, would diminish the strength of the white race. These allegations continued even after Chinese immigration was effectively halted through the Exclusion Act of 1882. Their echo was heard in the SARS scare just a few years ago.

Similarly, in the 1890s and early 1900s, Italian and Eastern European Jewish immigrants in New York were accused not only of bringing polio and tuberculosis, respectively, but of degrading American civilization with their hereditary mental and physical defects—claims that came not only from among the uneducated but from professors at prominent universities. Intensive medical inspections allowed authorities at Ellis Island to turn back would-be immigrants who were seen as socially undesirable by alleging that they had TB, trachoma of the eye, or other contagious conditions.

Italian immigrants were indeed more likely than native-born New Yorkers to die of measles and diarrhea (associated with poverty and crowding) at that time, but they were less likely to die of polio. And in 1910, New York State residents who had been born in Russia, most of whom were probably Jews, were almost 50 percent less likely than native-born citizens whose parents were also native-born to die of tuberculosis. Allegations that the new strangers were germ carriers were not borne out by the data.

The assumption that foreign status equaled germiness was a powerful force, as was the notion that disease susceptibility signaled racial inferiority. Some people demanded special control of the suspect populations—controls ostensibly against disease but really against supposedly germ-carrying immigrants. These demands put native-born Americans who shared the immigrants' heritage in a curious position, especially when disease did break out among immigrants. When destitute Russian Jews arrived in America in great numbers in the 1890s, after a series of oppressive policy moves and murderous pogroms against Jews directed by the czar, they were accused of causing two outbreaks of contagion (first typhus and then cholera) in New York. The German Jews of an earlier generation of immigrants were put in a deeply ambivalent position—the bind of what writer Richard Goldstein has called implication and immunity. Medical historian Howard Markel has found that, on the one hand, they were disdainful of the new immigrants: the newcomers seemed to be un-

educated peasants and laborers, speaking Yiddish and Russian but neither German nor English, and sharing little of the high culture to
which the German Jews aspired. In particular, second-generation Jewish New Yorkers had to worry that allowing themselves to be linked
with the first-generation arrivals might blemish their reputation as
dependable, assimilated members of middle-class America. On the
other hand, to permit disease outbreaks to ravage their coreligionists
would invite nativists and anti-Semites alike to tar the German Jews
with the same brush that painted the Russian Jews as engines of
degradation. The native-born Jews had to take action to avoid implication. They raised funds for social improvement and health care for
Jewish immigrants at the same time as they lobbied federal officials
not to blame cholera on immigrants.

In 1900, an outbreak of plague in San Francisco associated with
that city's Chinatown put Chinese Americans in an even more pre-
carious position. When a forty-one-year-old Chinese immigrant
businessman died of plague, the city's Board of Health ordered Chinatown cordoned off from the rest of the city. The police isolated about
fifteen square blocks, penning roughly 25,000 Chinese residents inside; only Caucasians were allowed to leave the isolation zone. At first
the Six Companies, a benevolent society for Chinese Americans,
urged their constituents to cooperate with health authorities. But after more plague cases were found, the authorities demanded that Chinese residents undergo inoculation with the experimental Haffkine
anti-plague vaccine, even though Haffkine recipients had experienced serious adverse effects in previous programs. American minds
so readily linked plague predisposition with Asian "race" that Japanese Americans were also required to undergo inoculation. And a hue
and cry arose that resonated with sentiments of the Black Death era:
there were calls to burn down Chinatown, and a plan was put forth
to replace the rope cordon with which Chinatown had been isolated
with a fence or a wooden wall. When many Chinese refused to sub-
mit to Haffkinization and business groups decried the effects of this

discriminatory policy on trade, Chinese Americans brought suit. In the *Jew Ho v. Williamson* decision, the Federal District Court in San Francisco found it impermissible to quarantine a national group without regard to whether individuals within that group were infectious. But while the case made it impossible to direct quarantines against an ethnic group, it hardly ended the practice of conflating foreignness with epidemic risk.

The episode of "Typhoid Mary" Mallon, an Irish cook in New York who was a healthy carrier of disease-causing bacteria, is well known. Mallon spread typhoid through her work in the kitchens of New York's upper classes. She is thought to be responsible for multiple outbreaks of typhoid, a severe diarrheal disease, in and around New York City between 1900 and 1915; several people died in the outbreaks associated with her. The city's health officials had Mallon isolated forcibly on North Brother Island in the East River. She spent a total of twenty-six years in isolation on this small island. Quite possibly, she would have been treated more benignly had she not been Irish and working class. But as it was, she was an implicit transgressor because she was of foreign and impoverished origins, and she was an explicit aggressor because she infected wealthy Americans.

GERMS, FLU, AND FEAR

By about 1910, germs had been shown to live in dust, the droplets of spit emitted when people talk, and the secretions left on human hands when they touch noses or eyes. That meant that germs could reside also on the things people touch—doorknobs, paper money, dishes, etc. Research revealed that microbes could be carried by insects, too; the body louse was by then known to spread the typhus microbe, a tick to carry Rocky Mountain spotted fever, mosquitoes to bear the germs of malaria and yellow fever, and the rat flea's bite to transmit plague. Germs were everywhere: they could crawl or fly onto people, or be ingested in food or drink. Constant vigilance was needed to keep them at bay. The path to health was to embrace new middle-class mores: keep houses and clothes clean, use new products and devices to combat dirt and dust, shave off beards that could harbor bacteria, seek medical care from doctors who use "scientific" techniques like antiseptics, and so forth. Americans still saw moral improvement as essential to avoiding illness, but they no longer thought of the moral imperative in terms of piety alone. Now it involved keeping clean.

By the First World War, with the findings of the microbiology revolution to draw on, germs were no longer only seeds of life, as Goethe thought of them, but the seeds of disease. In America, proper behavior became key to avoiding germs. Progressives, emphasizing purity of deed and spirit as ways to ward off contagion, put germs to a social use, recoding disease as an expression of character. The filth that clung to the lower classes was not only squalid and distasteful, in Progressive eyes, but also dangerous. If cleanliness meant the absence of germs (it didn't, but it would have seemed so as antisepsis and then sterilization made hospitals look clean), then dirtiness meant germiness. Special fears of dust and dirt, where germs were presumed to lurk, contributed. Dread of both unseen forces and the unpredictability of nature could be invested in germs—especially since germs are never visible to the unaided eye, and therefore their action could never be anticipated. Germs allowed the affluent to explain why the poor, in their unwashed garments, seemed so distasteful: they were *infected.*

—⚮—

Germ theory might never have become available to support suspicions about the indigent, foreigners, or despised races were it not for flu. The vast outbreak of influenza of 1918–1919, the so-called Spanish Flu, was the deadliest disease event the world has known. In a little over a year, Spanish Flu killed 20 million, or 40 million, or 50 million people worldwide. Although there are many estimates, the true number of casualties is unknown, because so many died where disease surveillance was rudimentary or simply too suddenly to allow for official tallies. In the United States, the number of deaths from Spanish Flu was about 550,000—roughly 0.5 percent of the population. That is the equivalent of about 1.5 million deaths in America today. The Spanish Flu outbreak cemented the germ as the pre-eminent threat to public health and gave to the microbe a leading role in the new concept of an epidemic.

The Spanish Flu might have scotched germ theory altogether, because germ theory was of so little help during the outbreak. Traditional precautions against epidemic illness still worked, up to a point, even those approaches that had been developed before any coherent scientific theory of germs had been formulated. Cities that isolated the sick and prevented people from congregating seemed to have somewhat lower mortality rates in the United States, for instance. But the great microbiologists and infectious-disease doctors were unable to do much to prevent the extensive mortality. Neither the new theory about microbes nor advances in lab technique enabled germ scientists to account for flu's sudden virulence or for the outbreak's global reach. Germ theory could not explain the unusual W-shaped pattern of mortality, with death rates high among people under five and over sixty-five years of age, as is typical for infectious outbreaks—but also among those ages twenty-five to thirty-five.

Scientific perplexity combined with wartime political demands accounted for the catastrophe's name. Flu outbreaks had begun among American, British, French, and German troops fighting in France and Belgium in the spring of 1918, and then struck Spain. Newspaper articles on flu appeared in Spanish papers because, as Spain was neutral in the war, it did not censor its press as the warring nations did. The relative absence of flu news from newspapers other than those in Spain, scientists' inability to locate its origins, and the traditional bent for attributing the source of epidemic disease to foreign lands allowed the outbreak to be labeled "Spanish." By the time the epidemic was first mentioned in New York papers, in mid-August 1918, it was already being called "Spanish influenza."

Influenza virus is transmitted very simply, by airborne droplets, and moves quickly from person to person. The virus changes its outer coat every year, just enough to be able to escape the human body's immune surveillance—so unlike measles, flu infection confers no lasting immunity. The phenomenon of changing its coat is called *antigenic drift*. Because of drift, effective influenza surveillance can be accomplished only by isolating the virus continually from people who get sick and checking on the specific makeup of the parts of the virus that elicit human immune response. This, in turn, allows disease-control planners to know exactly how to create each year's flu vaccine. Occasionally, though, the flu virus undergoes a more dramatic genetic change called *antigenic shift*, which renders flu capable of causing widespread illness with high mortality—this is what happened in 1918.

On the individual level, an uninfected person can protect herself from flu by staying home until all the infected people in her community have recovered (or died). Transmission of flu virus between people who are not normally in close contact happens primarily in settings of great crowding and poor ventilation. While it might not be practicable for people to remain cloistered in their homes, banning large gatherings, shutting schools or public transportation, or disbanding army camps can slow the virus's spread. This is exactly what happened in 1918. But flu is simply too easy to communicate, too likely to cause illness once infection occurs, and too readily coughed or sneezed outward by those who are sick to be easy to control at the population level. Not much can be done about flu's public-health harms, unless a vaccine is available—and there was none in 1918.

By 1918, after a couple of decades of rising popularity, germ theory seemed to signal the imminent control of disease. When the American Museum of Natural History in New York mounted its "Garden of Germs" exhibit of the causative agents of many important diseases in

1917, it implied that microbes could be captured, tamed, and stuffed. In so confident a milieu, the horror of the 1918 flu should have awak-ened grave skepticism about the value of germ theory in public health. Instead, the epidemic seemed to consolidate germ theory's power, corroborating the sense that germs signal impending catastro-phe and validating the worst fears that germ theory awoke: the dread that we are vulnerable to invasion by an invisible "army" of secret agents and indiscernible carriers. (Evidence now suggests that the United States was not invaded by Spanish Flu at all; it might have been a homegrown American product, the genetic recombination by which a garden-variety flu virus becomes one of those strains that can produce a lethal global outbreak possibly having taken place on farms in America's midsection.)

Testament to the force of germ theory to awaken innate anxieties about nature, the 1918 flu remains exhibit A when people seek to frighten us about potential virus-borne catastrophe today. Evidence came in the form of the swine flu affair, a 1976 federal campaign to immunize every American against a strain of flu that was, supposedly, identical to the 1918 strain. The effort ended, after only 45 million Americans had been immunized, because of a near-complete absence of cases of illness caused by the supposedly recrudescent flu strain and the possibility that the immunization induced an ascending paralysis called Guillain-Barré syndrome in hundreds of vaccine recipients. The U.S. government paid out nearly $93 million in legal settle-ments and lost judgments to claimants who said they had been in-jured by the vaccine.

Today evidence of germ theory's continuing capacity to give voice to unreasoning fear is the reaction to avian flu. It is a strain of influenza virus that began causing illness among birds in the Far East in the 1990s. Eighteen human cases of flu caused by the same H5N1 strain of bird-influenza virus were reported in Hong Kong in 1997, and human cases began to appear in China in 2003. As avian flu has continued to spread through bird flocks, it has also continued to throw off occasional human infections—by the autumn of 2008 there had been more than 380 human cases in total, about 60 percent of them fatal. The potential for any sustained outbreak among humans seems small, though. This particular flu virus evidently acquired the ability to infect people early on, but over ten years and millions of bird deaths, it has caused human illness only rarely. When humans are exposed to infected poultry, they are not infected at high rates. North American migratory birds are not very susceptible to the highly pathogenic subtypes of the avian flu virus, which would seem to limit the potential for spread in the Western Hemisphere and thus for any pandemic of the 1918 sort. Most important, humans do not spread the virus to other humans. Despite the poor prospects that H5N1 flu might create a serious human outbreak, scientists and officials have invoked the Spanish Flu scenario to demand resources for pandemic-flu planning. They use the fears embedded in germ theory to persuade us to keep financing their research, pay for their virus-detection or virus-prevention products, and use tax money for flu-preparedness exercises.

Based on the elegant scientific work of a team that reconstituted the influenza strain responsible for the 1918–1919 epidemic (which is different from the avian flu strain), it now appears that a very small number of genetic changes could turn an animal flu virus into a disease-causing agent for humans, with the capacity to produce local outbreaks. Could today's avian flu undertake such a journey to create a human disease event on a global scale? Nobody can predict whether local human outbreaks, even if they do occur, would become widespread. We know little about the resistance of human populations to H5N1 flu viruses. For instance, it seems possible that in the parts of the world most likely to allow for a bird-to-human jump on the part of the virus, many people might be resistant to H5N1 flu strains because of prior exposure (widespread immunity to H5N1 influenza would act as a damper on a human epidemic, if one were to occur). There is at least a little epidemiologic evidence that such resistance exists in China, one of the places where such a jump might be likely.

Treatment with antiviral drugs, if implemented immediately after symptoms begin, would also damp human-to-human spread of H5N1 flu by reducing the duration of infectivity. Concern has been voiced over the avian flu strain's ability to resist antiviral medications. But medical virologists know a lot about medicating people infected with highly mutable viruses. Combination therapy, that is, using more than one antiviral drug at a time, might be effective even if the virus becomes resistant to one or another medication singly.

Even if avian flu becomes capable of human-to-human spread, the genetic changes that would be required to allow it to move from person to person might not be stable. Without a persistent genetically programmed capacity to maintain both infectivity and pathogenicity for humans, the H5N1 virus could produce focal human outbreaks but not a pandemic like that seen in 1918.

Today, unlike in 1918, we have both hindsight—we know how bad a flu pandemic can be—and advance warning of new flu strains and where they strike. Unlike in 1918, we command considerable knowledge of the workings of the influenza virus, and we know how to immunize against it. Vaccines do not need to be 100 percent effective to be useful in protecting the public. Even a partially effective vaccine—one that successfully immunizes a majority of the population but does not protect everyone—can prevent a serious epidemic if it is carefully and sensibly administered in susceptible populations. Technology, that is, will help. The public-health apparatus has been very effective at limiting outbreaks of infectious disease.

THE AFTERMATH OF GERM THEORY

Fearmongering wasn't invented by germ scientists, nor was it the main intent of physicians who sought to use scientific findings about bacteria and viruses to forestall the advance of infectious illnesses like TB, typhoid, or flu. But germ theory changed the way the story of imminent epidemic cataclysm is told. The prefatory phase of an epidemic, the time when not much seems to be happening, can now be understood as a latent period: the hidden germs are percolating through the population but not yet manifest. Therefore, even when nothing seems to be happening, fear-spreaders can claim that germs might be incubating. The signals can be sensed—and therein lies the importance of the connection between germs and morality. The harbingers of impending contagion, the rhetoric goes, are evident in morally tinged aspects of social life: in the mixing of sexes and races, the growth of cities (where both sorts of mixing might occur), sexual license, or the use of alcohol or drugs. What might seem like a loosening of traditional strictures holds the seed of imminent disaster. When people are doing something that seems risky, germs might be on the loose, ready to ignite disaster.

The misuse of germ theory to incite anxiety or shake loose some funding, and the appropriation of germs to craft narratives about human dread, don't mean that the science behind microbial pathogenesis of human disease is wrong. In the long run, germ theory has helped modern human society deal with many forms of contagious disease, flu not least among them. We now have the capacity to create effective vaccines that limit illness and mortality, tailored to each new strain of flu that comes around, having "drifted" immunologically from that of the preceding year. Immunization, against flu as well as numerous other transmissible infectious diseases, is one of the great public-health benefits of germ theory. Vaccination predated germ theory by about a century, but it took the resolve provided by the "one germ, one disease" approach to turn the method originally improvised by Edward Jenner to stop smallpox into a technique that is useful against many viruses. The certainty that wiping out a germ would wipe out the illness it caused allowed for the implementation of immunization across the board and helped to create the political will to immunize a great many people, so that certain infections could be rendered unthreatening. Smallpox had been eliminated from the face of the earth by 1978, through an international effort that involved no social reform or economic miracle, just laborious delivery of vaccine to every nook and cranny and painstaking administration to every susceptible person. Polio immunization made its debut in 1955 and has since allowed the transmission of naturally occurring poliovirus to be stopped in the United States (there are still cases of polio because of rare "leakage" of infectious virus from the vaccine preparation). One day soon, polio will be extinct globally. In the United States, broad-scale immunization has eliminated domestic transmission of measles and rubella viruses. They will also, one day, be extinct. A new vaccine against human papillomavirus holds the potential to diminish dramatically the occurrence of cancers of the cervix, penis, and anus.

Germ theory also lent itself to the enterprise of improving public health. It has allowed public-health officials to refine the old-fashioned contagion-control techniques, making them more effective—as the SARS episode demonstrated. It has guided the building of containment systems for those germs that cannot be suppressed with immunization: filters that keep air from becoming contaminated in labs and hospitals, antiseptics that keep food-service facilities from spreading pathogens, antibiotics that not only relieve the suffering of people with bacterial infections but break the transmission cycles that allow those bacteria to spread. Germ theory has had its uses.

But the downsides of germ theory are considerable, even apart from its co-option by doomsayers. Our wholehearted embrace of germ theory has been at the expense of subtlety of explanation—especially a loss of nuance in locating the roots of disease in the complexity of social conditions. The miasmatists might have had the details wrong when they thought foul-smelling air could carry illness, but they were right that understanding where disease breaks out, and who gets it, requires an attention to the specific circumstances of life in human society. The detail that the miasmatists missed was crucial, but the context they sought to supply was crucial, too.

Naturally, there is a push to circumscribe germ theory with social and environmental context. Epidemiologists of the late twentieth cen-

tury talked about the "web of causation" and "eco-epidemiology"—
meaning that the supposedly universal laws that determine how and
when disease occurs arise from interacting systems. These were noble
efforts to expand the scope of theorizing about the cause of disease
from the very particular germ to the more general ecosystem. But they
changed little. Perhaps they failed because they were wedded to the
flabby notion that science proceeds historically, as a progression from
one all-encompassing "paradigm" (that is, a way of thinking about nature) to the overthrow of that paradigm and adoption of a new one.
This was never a good description of what happens in science. Perhaps
the attempts to broaden the purview of epidemiology beyond germs to
ecosystems foundered precisely because the germ theory was not wrong
and therefore can't be thrown out. Germ theory isn't incorrect; it's just
misleading.

Depictions of epidemic disease have become simple in the germ-
theory era: when epidemiologists try to understand specifically how
infections spread, they rely on mathematical models that require
them to name a limited set of variables as relevant to outbreaks (for
instance, the intrinsic infectivity of the virus, what proportion of the
population was previously infected, how much natural resistance
people might harbor, the so-called survival function predicting
length of life under different circumstances, and the rates at which
people migrate in or out of the population of interest). And epidemiologic model makers use these quantities to reduce the complex natural system within which the disease outbreak occurs to a series of
equations. This makes for exciting math and, properly handled, allows for the framing of some scientific hypotheses that can be tested
by real-world observation. Adding "interacting systems" like climate
or race, which is the point of eco-epidemiologic models, makes the
mathematics more complicated and doesn't alter the fundamental inability of rigid concepts about how disease is produced to account for
the nuance and unpredictability of disease outbreaks in the real
world. Mathematical models give us "superspreaders," but they do
not tell us what conjunction of conditions enables one person to

spread virus efficiently and another not at all. Mathematical models strip disease of its imponderables: why some societies suffer more, how to explain different rates of illness in two neighborhoods that seem similar, why disease spreads faster in some seasons than others. In effect, germ theory answers a call. It focuses our dreads and provides the packages: the bacillus, the spirochete, the virus, etc. They are well described by laboratory scientists (we can even see photographs), and the circumstances under which they can be killed or their reproduction stopped are well understood. But if we were not so keen on attributing the cause of each outbreak of contagion to a germ, we might not see microbes as devil's messengers or configure the epidemic as an outrage or punishment.

CHAPTER 5

THE CONQUEST OF CONTAGION

A tropical entropy seemed to prevail, defeating grand schemes even as they were realized. Minor drug deals took place beneath the then unfinished people-mover tracks . . . and plans were under way for yet another salvage operation . . . a twenty-eight-acre sports arena and convention hall that could theoretically be reached by either Metrorail or people mover and offered the further advantage, since its projected site lay within the area sealed off during the 1982 Overtown riot, a district of generally apathetic but occasionally volatile poverty, of defoliating at least twenty-eight acres of potential trouble.

—JOAN DIDION, *MIAMI*, 1987

By late 2002, a year after the postal anthrax event, "bioprepared-ness" was on the national tongue in America. A November 2002 CDC publication (no longer available) recommended immunization of a million so-called first responders. In December, President George W. Bush announced a plan to protect Americans against smallpox, although the last time an American had been stricken with smallpox was in 1949 and the disease was defunct by 1978. The federal government was planning to immunize half a million armed-forces personnel and another half-million civilians against an extinct disease.

The government's rationale was that rogue scientists might have taken samples of deep-frozen smallpox virus from labs in the former Soviet Union and sold them to terrorists. Or perhaps the scientists themselves had gone to work for terrorist organizations. They might have thawed the smallpox samples, tinkered with the genes, and weaponized the germs. The explanations about scientists' penchant for messing with nature and the presumptively ghastly results were disturbingly reminiscent of 1950s science-fiction films like *Them!* (1954) or *Attack of the Crab Monsters* (1957), which featured enormous ants and nasty crabs that had been produced by nuclear testing.

The first responders did not come forward for smallpox immunization. By late January 2003 only one U.S. state had begun a serious vaccination program, and the vaccination campaign fizzled. By February 2003 the footprints of the original plan had been removed from federal Web sites, leaving only the bare bones of a recommendation for immunization of "smallpox response teams." Through years of seemingly unceasing talk of a "war on terror," no foreigners troubled the health of America's cities, office parks, mail rooms, or football stadiums.

PROGRESSIVISM AND MORALISM

In the germ era, the plot of the traditional epidemic story took on a new twist. After the epidemic had run its course, things only *seemed* to be returning to normal. The germs might have gone to ground, found a hiding place, or been taken up by "rogue scientists." They were tiding themselves over, and they might rise again. On the last page of Camus's *The Plague*, the narrator tells us that "the plague bacillus never dies or disappears for good . . . it can lie dormant for years and years in furniture and linen-chests . . . it bides its time in bedrooms, cellars, bunks, and bookshelves; and . . . it would rouse up its rats again and send them forth to die in a happy city." That germs might leave and return was apparent after the experience of repeat attacks of plague from the 1340s to the 1600s and of cholera in the 1800s. That they might linger, present but unrecognizable as a constant risk, was a thought spurred by new anxieties. Fears of industrial pollution, social upheaval, and sexual degeneracy—fears of modernity—easily translated into fear of germs.

If the city was a happy place, by the twentieth century it had become a suspect place, especially in America. With its hodgepodge of languages, nationalities, and callings and its potential for unexpected social and sexual intimacies, the city was the more repugnant when it seemed to be infused with germs.

Fear of germs was a strong force for social change. Progressive social reformers used germ theory to redefine sexually transmissible diseases, reshape medical practice, and revise sexual mores. In the United States, preventing contagion became a professed goal of Progressives whose main aim was to protect the stability of a new sort of American marriage. With awareness that the main venereal diseases (VD) of the industrial era, syphilis and gonorrhea, were microbe-borne, Progressive social reformers rallied to change sexual habits in the United States and Britain.

Both syphilis and gonorrhea had been around for many generations. Syphilis, which results from infection with the spiral-shaped bacterium *Treponema pallidum*, had been responsible for furious and sometimes deadly outbreaks when it first began to spread sexually in Europe, in the 1490s—either when an already circulating microbe acquired the capacity to be transmitted through sexual intercourse or when it was brought back to Europe from the New World on Spanish ships of exploration (the source remains controversial). Syphilis swept through Europe and eventually reached Japan by about 1505. As is commonly true with infectious pathogens, the virulence of syphilis declined over time, but through the late nineteenth century it remained a severe condition that could lead to death from cardiovascular or nervous-system maladies. Gonorrhea, caused by infection with the bacterium *Neisseria gonorrhoeae*, had probably been in circulation in

Western societies for even longer. Well before the nineteenth century, both had settled into a pattern of slow and continuous circulation.

Syphilis rates tend to cycle periodically—nowadays there are up-swings every decade or so, followed by downturns. These shifts might have occurred somewhat more slowly in the less mobile society of the nineteenth century. Gonorrhea rates change in less regular fashion. (The reasons for oscillations in VD rates remain mysterious even now, but it is obvious that incidence rates can change even when sexual habits do not.) Data on the real prevalence of syphilis and gonorrhea in the late nineteenth and early twentieth centuries are spotty, but both diseases were clearly common and had been on the rise since the mid-1800s. In England and Wales, for instance, the neonatal death rate from syphilis (*T. pallidum* can be passed from infected mother to developing fetus) had risen from about 1,200 newborn deaths per million live births in 1854–1867 to about 1,700 per million in 1868–1898. Around 1910, 2 percent of U.S. servicemen were admitted to hospitals for venereal conditions and about 10 percent of all Americans were estimated to have syphilis. Beyond the acute effects of VD on the sufferers, considerable associated morbidity, including infertility and congenital blindness in the newborn, caused medical concern.

Even today, when we know that syphilis rates can go up independently of changes in sexual behavior, U.S. health officials warn Americans about sexual behavior and responsibility. What aroused reformers' attention at the end of the nineteenth century and the first years of the twentieth was that the increases in rates of the long-established conditions coincided with scientists' demonstration that VD was germ-borne. The conjunction of rising VD rates, knowledge of germs, and desire to reform sex roles in modern society created new concerns about how sexual behavior was tied to social status.

Progressives responded by working to dispel the traditional belief that innate and irremediable sexual drives commanded men to "sow wild oats." They argued for male continence instead. To support the change in habits, Progressives demanded widespread sex education, particularly because they thought the working classes were more easily led into allegedly perverse and dangerous sexual habits, that is, premarital and extramarital sex. They would teach men to forswear sexual relationships with women other than their wives. To induce husbands to be sexually faithful, as wives traditionally had been expected to be, marriage would be promoted as the central source of intimacy and emotional nurturance for both parties. Once the companionate marriage had become the standard of the middle and upper classes, it would be emulated by the laboring classes, eager for upward mobility. The new, more stringent fidelity of American marriages could be promoted not only as a moral good and as a hedge against divorce but also as a preventive against the threat of venereal disease, which would reduce, in turn, stillbirth and congenital defects in the marriage's offspring. In this way, Progressives turned sexual licentiousness into an assault on the health of future generations.

The crusade against VD made room for activists seeking gender equality, those advocating sexual propriety, and physicians who saw reducing VD transmission as a medical obligation. Doctors came to espouse Progressive sexual moralism, while social activists embraced germ control to stop VD. The social reformers claimed that marriage would benefit from this equalizing, and venereal disease rates would fall. Forming the American Society for Sanitary and Moral Prophylaxis in 1905, social hygienists worked to combat the spread of contagion that was rooted in "social evil" (that is, sex).

Medical practice changed as a result. When American doctors allied their own anti-VD work with the social-hygiene movement's campaign to improve marriage, some felt obligated to impart to wives information on their husbands' infection with syphilis or gonorrhea— divulging what had once been a secret kept by husbands in collusion with their doctors. And in some cases the doctors' professed aim was to halt the allegedly degrading effects of VD on the white race.

In the policy realm, the social-hygiene campaign took the form of crackdowns on prostitution and laws requiring screening for syphilis before marriage. The persuasive rationale of disease control gave new meaning to official policies that suppressed sex work as a buttress to the new model of marriage and sexual propriety. Prostitutes were already stigmatized in America on moral grounds before scientists determined that venereal diseases were the result of microbial infections. But moral reproof alone meant that a woman was a danger only to herself if she took money for sex (or, really, if she was lustful). Once people believed that a woman who sold sex carried germs, they could claim that she was dangerous to everyone. By association, sex work was presumed to be its own kind of moral germ. Social hygienists thought that some women in the sex trade had started out virtuous but, infected with syphilis or gonorrhea pathogens by indiscreet husbands, descended into harlotry.

Progressive crusaders also saw a connection between sex work and factory work in America's cities, and some associated labor in manufacturing plants with the decline of the American family. In part, this imagined connection reflected the subtle influence of the Jeffersonian vision of America, by which the agrarian life was the healthy life. But in part it was also based on economics: industrial workers were subject to occasional layoffs; therefore, the modernization of manufacturing, which drew young women out of homes and into the urban workforce, also encouraged them to stave off penury when they were unemployed by selling their bodies. Whether there was truth to this assumption seems to have been less important to the reformers than that it plausibly created a rationale for looking suspiciously at the modern city. In Progressive eyes, the bacteria responsible for the two prominent sexual infections were threats to American health, genetic soundness, and morality. Prostitution had to be suppressed as a source and outcome of these perils, and the urban laborer needed both health improvement and moral guidance. The quest for immunity from infection was not far from the quest for purity.

To constrain male sexual incontinence, the Progressive moral campaign created a duty on the part of men to protect the purity of women by avoiding germs. For instance, the U.S. Army's Social Hygiene Division appealed to soldiers in the First World War to return "physically fit and morally clean," with posters showing images of neatly dressed women and children in home settings who, by implication, might be infected if the troops were to bring home VD. By the Second World War, posters and training films for American troops depicted "loose women," "good-time girls," and "pick-ups" who might look "clean" but were dangerous. The appeal had shifted, but the moral valence was the same: women who are sexual are dangerous; women who are pure deserve protection. Explicitly, it is venereal contagion from which the soldier is meant to protect the womenfolk back home by avoiding the foreign prostitute. Implicitly, it is immorality that he must keep at bay (see figures 5 and 6).

Avoidance of epidemic VD became part of the rationale for reinforcing the moral viewpoint that sexual correctitude is a social responsibility in the social-hygiene era. The term "social hygiene" transparently came to mean "sexual probity." The social-hygiene movement did have decidedly beneficial results, raising awareness about sexually transmissible infection as a hazard to public health, instating sex education as an institution in schools, and opening the public conversation about sex. But the first sexual revolution did little to alter American disapproval of women's sexual license.

Continental Europe was also beleaguered in the early twentieth century by sexually transmissible infections and illness. In France and Germany, authorities instituted a policy of *reglementation*, strictly regulating sex work and requiring periodic medical inspection of women who sold sex—a more effective method for limiting the damage caused by genital infections than American penalization of sex work. Although some American physicians and a few vice officers in U.S. cities considered similar approaches, *reglementation* ran counter to American Progressivism. As the historian Allan Brandt points out, American purity crusaders sought continence from both sexes. Still, while regulatory approaches to prostitution were less morally tinged, interpreting microbial infection as a sign of moral deficiency was strong in Europe. Franz Kafka, writing to his ex-fiancée, Felice Bauer, sometime after he was diagnosed with TB in 1917, said, "Secretly I don't believe this illness to be tuberculosis, at least not primarily tuberculosis, but rather a sign of my general bankruptcy."

GERMS AND THE SEXUAL REVOLUTION

The notion that sexual women were germ carriers continued to undergird anxieties about female sexuality even after the middle of the twentieth century. Syphilis and gonorrhea were brought under some control with antibiotic treatment and through the public-health intervention of contact tracing.* But when rates of new diagnoses of syphilis and gonorrhea began to increase dramatically and continued rising through the 1970s, it was easy to blame the advent of the birth-control pill or "promiscuity," the hallmarks of the sexual revolution of the 1960s. The declining age of onset of intercourse and increasing premarital sexual experience were real, but they had undergone more of an evolution than a revolution, and they probably had little to do with climbing rates of syphilis and gonorrhea. Still, syphilis and gonorrhea became parts of speech in the dialogue about sexual revolution and the larger and lasting debates about the cultural changes of the era.

The supposed epidemic of VD in the 1960s and '70s was probably not much a consequence of changing behavior. Undeniably, contemporary culture was suddenly sexualized in many ways, including ad-

---

*Penicillin was first used in 1942, not against VD but in a case of streptococcal infection in New Haven, Connecticut. Shortly thereafter it was employed against syphilis and gonorrhea, first in the military and then generally, to good effect. Contact tracing is a public-health tool, in which health officers ask people treated for sexually transmissible infections to supply names and addresses of sexual contacts. Officials then visit the named contacts and offer them testing and treatment.

vertising, the entertainment industry, and everyday speech. There was greater tolerance for expressions of female desire and women having sex outside of marriage, even though the double standard by which men were admired for taking sexual license but women were deplored for it didn't disappear. There was also the beginning of a movement toward acceptance of same-sex coupling. But the increases in VD rates in that era are best explained by deeper social shifts and changes in public-health policy. Case detection and reporting improved as the stigma of diagnosis with a genital infection declined. In the United States, the expanding heterogeneity of social interactions, increased mobility, and extension of higher education to broader segments of the population allowed for greater mixing among Americans of different backgrounds. New patterns of sexual partner choice allowed VD to escape from the subsets of the population where it had been concentrated, becoming more broadly prevalent. At the same time, as sometimes happens after initial success, federal spending for case finding, contact tracing, and control declined. Finally, natural fluctuations in the population size and infectivity of the two main bacteria in question, *T. pallidum* and *N. gonorrhoeae*, always allowing for ebb and flow in the way VD moves through the population, contributed to temporary increases at that time—ecological shifts that had nothing to do with sexual behavior.

Even though complex forces contributed to rising syphilis and gonorrhea rates, in the last quarter of the twentieth century public-health professionals joined moralizing commentators to attribute newly surging contagion to the old standbys: improper behavior and the sex trade. In the 1980s and '90s, the CDC repeatedly issued reports, based on small-area studies and investigations of outbreaks of syphilis or gonorrhea, implicating prostitution, even where the data collected didn't pertain to professional commercialized sex per se but individuals' personal accounts of having exchanged sex for either money or drugs. Official reports on sexual contagion in that era implied that female sexual behavior is inherently hazardous.

"YOU CANNOT HAVE OMELETTES
WITHOUT BREAKING EGGS"

As it has been easy for Western men to presume that the female body, in sexual congress or merely in a state of desire, is unclean, so too have Western societies seen threats in the bodies of the poor and dark. European countries with a history of colonialism seem to have been particularly susceptible to myths of congenital uncleanness on the part of foreigners.

Early in the nineteenth century, when James Mill sought to rationalize British economic takeovers in India, he claimed that Indian society would never escape its primitiveness. By the century's end, both British and French colonialists had made similar claims about Africans, couched in the language of disease. Africans were supposed to be constitutionally incapable of advancement. Malaria, leprosy, yellow fever, and schistosomiasis were taken to be signs of their biological incapacity to ward off disease. The founder of the Yellow Fever Bureau at the London School of Hygiene and Tropical Medicine wrote in 1911 that West Africans are "lowly organized human beings" and that Europeans who first ventured there "found themselves face to face with a . . . veritable pack of children." Ronald Ross, the Scottish physician credited with discovering that anopheline mosquitoes transmit malaria, wrote from Sierra Leone that "the native . . . is really nearer a monkey than a man." From the late 1800s until at least the 1920s, members of the medical establishment assumed that Africans and their descendants were hereditarily immune to malaria and yellow fever, even as the infectious nature of both diseases came to be accepted. The concept of racial immunity offered a pseudoscientific rationale for social and economic development of Africa, and a medical justification for racial subjugation—so much so that the field of tropical medicine was called "colonial medicine" in parts of Europe. Identifying and curing Africans of the germs that beleaguered them would provide a healthier labor force for the use of colonial administrators and would bring international prestige in the fields of science and medicine.

In the social Darwinist milieu, germ theory gave race theorists a card to play both ways. On the one hand, they could interpret infection within African populations as evidence of hereditary susceptibility, which meant lesser fitness. On the other hand, low disease rates were also grounds for race-theory interpretation, allegedly showing that those who failed to get sick were more primitive. In the inherited-susceptibility view, schistosomiasis (a parasitic infection acquired by bathing in contaminated waters) and trypanosomiasis (sleeping sickness, whose causative parasite is transmitted by the tsetse fly) were grounds for wide-scale economic-development campaigns British and Belgian colonizers forced on Africans—the stated aim being to provide the "civilizing" institutions that the Africans were too congenitally weak to create themselves. Under the primitive-race view, the low frequency of yellow fever among adults in parts of West Africa (where infants and small children infected with the yellow fever virus tended to have mild or inapparent illness and remained immune thereafter, keeping rates low) was understood as proof that heredity kept the more primitive orders immune while the more advanced—European whites—developed susceptibility.

Predisposition to epidemic illness and immunity from it both hinged on race as a genetic entity, with biological concomitants. Both justified the colonizers' subjecting Africans to schemes for "improvement" that were at least as profitable to the rulers as they were beneficial to Africans' health. British colonial secretary Joseph Chamberlain warned in 1897 that developers might have to resort to force to uplift the West Africans, whom he characterized as barbaric and superstitious, famously remarking that "you cannot have omelettes without breaking eggs."

Construing higher disease rates as emblems of racial inferiority helped drive political developments in Europe. In France, medical authorities in the 1910s urged that syphilis diagnosis and treatment be instituted, lest the white race degenerate. Under the Third Reich, Germany went a step further, configuring syphilis as a threat to race purity. The program was attractive not only to ideologues and race theorists but also to many medical professionals. By 1939 the journal *Ziel und Weg*, founded just before Hitler's takeover to carry articles on race medicine, had become the preeminent voice of Nazi race philosophy on health and had a readership of more than 40,000. The Genetic Health Courts (*Erbgesundheitsgerichte*) administered a National Socialist government program that forcibly sterilized people who had so-called genetic diseases, including schizophrenia, manic-depressive disorder, epilepsy, Huntington's chorea, "hereditary alcoholism," grave congenital physical malformation, congenital blindness, and congenital deafness. This list provided an excuse to sterilize perpetrators of "sex crimes" in general and VD carriers in particular, since malformations and visual defects can arise in a child born to a mother infected with syphilis or gonorrhea bacteria.

As frightening as it seems today, the German forced-sterilization program was modeled on well-articulated American eugenic principles. The law governing the Nazi sterilization program was drawn from the Model Sterilization Law drafted by Harry Laughlin, a prominent American eugenicist. Laughlin, who was expert eugenics agent for the House Committee on Immigration and Naturalization and later superintendent of the Eugenics Records Office at Cold Spring Harbor on Long Island, proposed a law by which a state would grant itself the right to sterilize. His law was enacted by the state of Virginia (and later elsewhere) and was carried out almost exclusively on poor, and disproportionately black, Americans. The law was vindicated in the 1927 *Buck v. Bell* Supreme Court decision. Upholding the right of states to sterilize the "unfit," Justice Oliver Wendell Holmes Jr. wrote for the Court's 8-to-1 majority that "it is better for all the world if . . . society can prevent those who are manifestly unfit from continuing their own kind. . . . Three generations of imbeciles are enough." In 1936, Harry Laughlin was honored by the Nazi government with an honorary doctorate.

The Nazi program's stunningly proactive approach to health promotion by linking race to infection and genetic pollution won acclaim well beyond Germany's borders. Articles in the *American Journal of Public Health* in 1934 and 1935 applauded the equitable administration of forcible sterilization through the Genetic Health Courts as well as the Nazi regime's capacity to instill in citizens a sense of responsibility for the public's health. One of those laudatory reports was written by the director of the U.S. National Tuberculosis Association, Dr. H. E. Kleinschmidt. American public-health experts ratified the choice of the nine genetic diseases that were grounds for compulsory sterilization in Germany and noted without comment that in a Berlin health exposition "the anti-Semitic policy is meticulously explained." They seem not to have noted the connections between contagion control and race medicine.

In 1939, the Nazi program expanded forcible sterilization into euthanasia to kill the genetically unsound. Nicknamed T4,* the euthanasia program was meant to cleanse the Aryan race of genetically damaging conditions by killing the mentally ill, including individuals with symptoms of late-stage syphilis. By 1941, T4 had exterminated 70,273 Germans labeled *lebensunwerten Lebens*, "worthless life." The murdered were not Jews or even foreigners; they were full-blooded Germans whose potential to breed additional generations of "defective" humans made them dangers to the Aryan *Volk.*

Scientific as it was supposed to sound, Nazi genetic hygiene was no more insulated from judgments of social behavior than the leprosy rules of the thirteenth century or the immigrant hysterias of the late nineteenth. The T4 program allowed for the extermination of

---

*It was administered from an office whose address was Tiergartenstrasse 4, in Berlin.

people who were deemed to be psychopaths only on the basis of out-sider (*gemeinschaftsfremd*, or "alien-to-the-community") criteria, such as prostitution, fraud, or homosexuality.

As practiced under the Third Reich, eugenics reified the con-nections among disease, hereditary purity, and race. Hitler had writ-ten that he felt like "Robert Koch in politics," uncovering the role of the "Jew as the bacillus." Equating the elimination of politically tainted peoples with preventing the propagation of unhealthy genes was a useful move: eugenics was exactly the metaphor by which the National Socialists made their Final Solution to the problem of "race defilement" (*Rassenschande*) seem reasonable. In 1941, when the large-scale extermination of Slavs, Jews, Gypsies, and other racial offenders became Reich policy, the T4 program simply melded into the broader program for racial cleansing that culminated in the extermination camps. By 1942, the Reich had approved euthanasia for Poles who had tuberculosis. The eugenic impulse to purify the race and the contagion-control policy of public health became in-distinguishable. Some of the same architects of T4 were transferred eastward, where they were involved directly in the Final Solution.

BEYOND EUGENICS

Genetic determinism is the old "seed and soil" explanation in modern guise. It makes room for race theories by finding evidence of heredi-tary inferiority in the spread of contagion. Genes are where the germ's potential lurks, it says. Hereditary susceptibility is fallow soil waiting for the errant germ to sprout an epidemic. Health officials today no longer dare to assert, as did Dr. Thomas Murrell (who would become a U.S. Public Health Service officer) in 1910, that "when diseased, [the Negro] should be forced to take treatment before he offers his diseased mind and body on the altar of academic and professional education." But officials still connect hereditary disease susceptibility to race. "Worthlessness," expunged from the modern public-health lexicon, lingers just behind our jargon of risk. When, in the name of disease control, our officials assert that people of African descent are especially susceptible to specific illnesses, they appeal to the same sensibility about race as a signal of genetic inferiority as did Murrell and the Nazi race theorists. Today, black Americans are said to be at higher risk of prostate cancer, infection with hepatitis B virus and HIV, and infant mortality, to name only a few health problems of concern. We do know what causes hepatitis B infection, and it is probably more common in African Americans for reasons that have to do solely with social clustering.* We do *not* know completely what causes prostate cancer or infant mortality; they are surely complex. Claiming that people of African descent are predisposed to such conditions explicitly attributes disease risk to genetics and implicitly attributes health to a person's fitness. And it ties fitness to race.

Racial theories of susceptibility to infection have harrowing historical resonances. Proponents of racial hygiene invoked images of infection to point up the alleged threat posed by the despised races. *Der Stürmer*, a propaganda organ for Nazi race policies, depicted Jews as the worm "Jewish Scandal" in the fruit of German economy in a 1931 cartoon (see figure 7). In the 1940 National Socialist propaganda film *Der ewige Jude (The Eternal Jew)*, rats teem while the voice-over reports that "where rats appear, they bring annihilation to the land . . . [rats] spread disease, plague, leprosy, typhus, cholera, dysentery, etc . . . just as Jews do among the people." Hitler not only referred to Jews as "bacilli" but also as "viruses" and "parasites," and he painted the Jewish population of the Soviet Union as a *Pestherd* (plague focus). Heinrich Himmler, in a speech to SS officers in Poznań (then the German city of

---

*A founder effect, in which the people most likely to acquire an infection and most likely to pass it on are those who are socially linked to the individuals who first contracted the infection, tends to sequester and amplify sexually transmitted and needle-borne infections like hepatitis B within small social groups.

Posen) in 1943, made plain the equation of Jews with bacteria: "In the end," he declaimed, "as we exterminate the bacillus, we wouldn't want to become sick with it and die [ourselves]."

—ɷ—

Racial hygiene and racial health gave new force to the old threat of syphilis. That syphilis can be transmitted from infected mother to developing fetus lent force to beliefs that it runs in the family as well as to suspicions that it might lurk undetected. But the disease had been around for centuries before a transmissible agent was identified, and it had long served the uses of xenophobes and moralists. Like most forms of contagion, syphilis was consistently attributed to outsiders. Unlike most other illnesses, though, syphilis allowed for sex to be connected explicitly with death, disfigurement, and dementia.

Still, until germ theory prompted the search for and discovery of the transmissible agent of syphilis, there was no clear causal story of syphilis from which to fashion a racial doctrine. *T. pallidum* was discovered in 1911, and the microbe was quickly promoted from infectious agent to cause of the disease. Before then, syphilis had been merely unspeakable. After that, Progressivism paired with germ theory. Once syphilis had entered the vocabulary of the social-hygiene dialogue, germs made syphilis a race matter.

However obvious it was that syphilis might affect anyone, regardless of social position, U.S. physicians in the first quarter of the twentieth century commonly believed that syphilis was different in black and white Americans. Common prejudices linking blackness to sexual depravity no doubt contributed to the assumption of difference. The mistaken belief that there are different genotypes neatly dividing the population into black and white served the further erroneous belief that the syphilis spirochete would behave differently in the "black" and "white" genetic settings and laid the foundation for the infamous Study of Untreated Syphilis in the Male Negro in Tuskegee, Alabama, in 1932.

Syphilis *was* highly prevalent among the impoverished African American dwellers of the rural South, no doubt partly because opportunities for schooling were few and partly because poor farmers, effectively indentured to the land they rented, could not afford medical care. Few clinics were open to black residents in that segregated region. In Macon County, Alabama, whose population was 82 percent black, a survey carried out by Dr. Taliaferro Clark of the U.S. Public Health Service (USPHS) reported that 36 percent of residents were infected with syphilis in 1929 and that 99 percent of those infected had never been treated. In the Study of Untreated Syphilis in the Male Negro, USPHS officials observed 199 men known to have syphilis but offered no treatment. Even after penicillin became the standard medical treatment for syphilis in the 1940s, USPHS officials who ran the study used private subterfuge and state power to ensure that treatment was denied the men under observation.

Well-known medical reports based on a series of men with syphilis in Oslo, Norway, had been published as recently as 1928 describing the course of untreated syphilis in men. Therefore, the Tuskegee syphilis "research" could not have been motivated by want of information on the course of syphilis. Only American physicians' refusal to believe that data on Norwegian white men could ever apply to American black men can explain how the USPHS justified the study medically in 1932. It is impossible to know if physicians really thought that syphilis could act differently in black people, or if this line of thinking was mere rationalization for looking at black Americans as less deserving. No moral justification could be adduced for the study in any case.

The Tuskegee study, which helped shape modern ideas about infection and race, was an egregious instance of the misuse of race in medicine. But it was neither the first nor the last time that immoral acts were committed against the disfavored in the name of medicine. Since 1972, when the Tuskegee study was exposed, many discussions of research ethics have charged the Tuskegee study investigators with conducting experiments without subjects' consent, without "equipoise," or with heartlessness born of racism. What is rarely spoken is that germs, especially germs that can be transmitted by sex, reinforce the separateness essential to the concept of race. To presume that it was reasonable, even necessary, to carry out research on a sexually transmitted germ among black Americans at a time when there was no clamor for further syphilis research on white Americans was to imply more than just that contagion is powerfully linked to genetic susceptibility—it implied that the behaviors necessary for the spread of contagion are themselves an aspect of the hereditary "soil" and make it more fertile for the disease-causing "seed." It signaled that race was a distinction that could be made by behavioral observation, because behavior was linked (somehow) to genetic predispositions.

The Tuskegee study could only have been undertaken and carried out for forty years because Americans' instincts toward disdaining sexual license and tendencies toward linking race to reprobate behavior drove more modern affinities for germs and genes. Neither lack of medical care nor inadequate treatment was seen as the root of the problem. Rather, it was black sexual habits that put the public in peril of infection. In 1910, when Dr. Thomas Murrell wrote that the mortal threats of syphilis and tuberculosis might together bring an "end of the negro problem," he meant that blackness implied inescapable tendencies toward dissolution and moral decline. And, he suggested, these tendencies would make deadly illness a certainty. Murrell was invoking the same principles that had fueled the eugenics of Ernst Haeckel and others a generation or more earlier. Germs might lurk within a race of people because their race made them act in ways that promoted infection.

European race myths connected blackness with syphilis, just as Americans' did. In 1917, when the American Expeditionary Force placed French brothels off-limits to U.S. troops, the mayor of St. Nazaire was especially concerned that black Americans with no sexual outlet would imperil local women, and he insisted either that brothels be opened for them or black women be imported from

America to provide sexual services. The Genetic Health Courts of the Third Reich, vigilant against potential damages to the Aryan gene pool, were directed in 1937 to order immediate sterilization of anyone who seemed to be of African ancestry.

American health advocates were more vigorous in pursuing the link between blackness and sexual infectiousness—not only in the sense that black people were assumed to be spreaders of sexually transmissible infections like syphilis but also by viewing black sexuality as licentious and threatening. The American eugenics advocate Dr. Harry Haiselden made a film in 1917 called *The Black Stork* to advertise the value of eliminating defective genes. In it, a wealthy white man is seduced by his black servant, producing half-caste progeny who ruin the well-bred family (see figure 8).

The American eugenics movement wound down after the Second World War, although it didn't die. The Nazi euthanasia program had evoked a generalized distaste for eugenic planning. And the availability of antibiotics to cure syphilis and gonorrhea undercut accusations that black syphilis carriers could imperil everyone. But the assumptions that black Americans were sexually dangerous merely changed form—or changed contagion: AIDS would later substitute neatly for syphilis as a shadow for white people to cast on darkskinned people, implying extraordinary sexual license and injudiciousness. The early attribution of AIDS's spread to Haitians would serve the same purpose, as would later discussions about HIV's origin in Africa. While it is almost undoubtedly true that HIV arose in Africa and first infected humans there, the "origin of AIDS" conversation would be heavily freighted with discussions of race and accusations of racism.

BEYOND GERM THEORY

Although the antibiotic penicillin was withheld from the men in the Tuskegee study, by midcentury it and other antibiotics began to show

their utility in limiting not only syphilis but other fearsome contagions. Antibiotics appeared to herald a new era in controlling once-
frightening communicable diseases like TB (it was a temporary
triumph, as the rise of antibiotic-resistant strains of TB, gonorrhea,
and other infections, now including the widely prevalent methicillin-
resistant *Staphylococcus aureus*, or MRSA, attest). Dramatic improvements in public health followed, in large measure because of the
embrace of the concept that each germ causes a disease. In America,
immunization furthered the gains made by administering antibiotics,
allowing smallpox to be eradicated after the last outbreak in 1947; polio to be curtailed dramatically in the '50s (domestic transmission was
finally eradicated in the '90s); and the contagious rashes that had
been common accompaniments of childhood, i.e., measles, mumps,
and rubella, to come under control in the 1960s (see page 139). In two
decades, measles vaccination alone saved 52 million Americans from
contracting the disease and spared more than 5,000 deaths. An international team conducted a campaign to eradicate smallpox with mass
vaccination. Beginning in the 1960s and ultimately transcending
even cold war constraints, the anti-smallpox campaign went on for
more than a decade and succeeded in eliminating the disease from the
face of the earth.

Germ theory's simple certainty about how to prevent epidemic
illness was a palliative for a world anxious about the capacity of disease threats to undo the stability and security it had earned by
weathering the war. And it offered a rationale by which can-do
leaders could view disease as just another enemy that needed to be
outgunned, a foe whom modern technology could subdue. The triumph of germ theory allowed a fearful public to believe that germs
were a constant threat yet also to feel secure that they could be conquered when they appeared.

The simplicity of germ theory provided direction to a new approach to epidemic control. Moving beyond the prevention of infectious threats, the postwar ideal was to do battle with epidemics in a

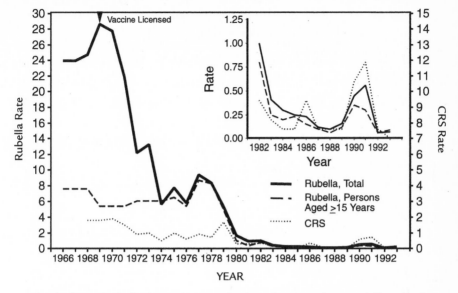

The decline of rubella ("German measles") in the United States following the implementation of vaccine in 1968. The vertical axis shows the number of annual cases per 100,000 population. *Source:* U.S. Centers for Disease Control and Prevention, "Rubella and Congenital Rubella Syndrome," *Morbidity and Mortality Weekly Report* 43, no. 21 (June 3, 1994): 397–401.

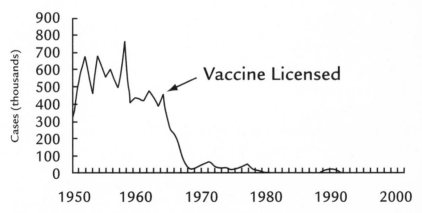

The rapid fall in U.S. measles incidence in the latter half of the twentieth century. The advent of vaccination against measles in 1963 produced a dramatic drop in the number of new cases each year. *Source:* U.S. Centers for Disease Control and Prevention, Vaccines & Immunizations Web site, at http://www .cdc.gov/vaccines/vac-gen/6mishome.htm#Diseaseshadalready (downloaded December 10, 2008).

broader sense. Investment expanded in research on the causes of non-infectious conditions like cancer, heart disease, and stroke, which had become prominent and, by the 1950s, had overwhelmed infections such as pneumonia, TB, and others as precipitants of death in industrialized countries. The simple model of prevention that germ theory provided, wherein disease is avoided by extirpating the single cause, proved to be applicable even when no germ was present. If the causes of the new epidemics could be identified, diseases could be stopped.

The disease arising from a single cause, by a simple pathway, easily became the culture's model in part because it offered a compellingly straightforward explanation for the mysteries of disease outbreaks. It thus reassured the residents of newly prosperous Western countries that their comfort would not be undone by epidemic illness. It resonated with the ideological wars of midcentury, the us-versus-them worldview in which nuance could be mere nuisance. In America, just when the industry of scientific research was expanding and looking for problems to study, the model suggested that eliminating the presumably simple causes of illness would be a worthy and practical goal for scientists. By the postwar years, there was technological firepower available to make the conquest of epidemics seem plausible if it was all as simple as germ theory proposed. Technological superiority made victory over the simple, germlike causes of illness seem not only theoretically possible but realistically within reach. Finally, moral imperatives demanded that everyone align their behavior with the hygienic norms of the middle classes so as to ward off dreadful contagions, which no longer seemed invincible. To engage the enemy became a civic duty.

The new view considered chronic conditions like cardiovascular problems and cancer, which threatened the well-being of the affluent, just as worrisome or more so than the communicable epidemics that imperiled the poor. It represented a shift in public health. Since germ theory served to alleviate the fears of the postwar world while continuing to offer a rationale for worries about race and sex, it is little surprise that it came to be the canonical story of the new public-health crusade that aimed to diminish threats to the comfort and longevity of the middle classes.

Another legacy of germ theory also worked in support of the "single cause, simple pathway" model, refashioning the way epidemics were viewed: germ theory gave the study of epidemics a *history*. What seemed to be true for physics, whose generally chaotic path toward apprehending the laws of nature was understood as being marked by the successive shifts in thought of Aristotle, Galileo, Newton, Watt, Einstein, and ultimately quantum mechanicians like Pauli and Heisenberg, could be claimed for epidemiology as well. This was an important claim for the new field of public health to be able to make, in support of its campaign to depict epidemic disease as a conquerable enemy. If public health was a march toward truth in much the way physics seemed to be, then the facts that mapped the fight against disease had the imprimatur of science. It became easier to build programs on the simple-seeming truths of single causes of disease—stop the influenza virus to prevent flu epidemics, stop smoking to prevent lung cancer. It also became easier to minimize the complicating truth: epidemics are events involving many interrelated aspects of an ecosystem of which germs, if they are involved at all, are merely one part. It was easier to muster popular will (and government funding) for the fight against germs, or against simple germlike causes of illness like smoking or dietary fat.

The position of science and scientists in the postwar struggle against natural threats to health was repeatedly illustrated in popular culture, perhaps most starkly in film. In Elia Kazan's Oscar-winning *Panic in the Streets*, a dedicated U.S. Public Health Service officer, played by Richard Widmark, tracks down criminals who have been exposed to a man carrying plague (not surprisingly a foreigner) and who might therefore spread the infection to the unsuspecting population of New Orleans. The public-health doctor must also keep his work secret because if residents find out, they might panic and flee, spreading plague to the rest of America. He succeeds, the selfless man of science saving an unknowing (and therefore ungrateful) population.

Science-fiction films repeated the theme: when a giant octopus imperils the city of San Francisco in Robert Gordon's 1955 thriller, *It Came from Beneath the Sea*, scientists rush to the rescue.

The "single cause, simple pathway" model was an essential ingredient of the so-called conquest of contagion. When Yale professor Charles-Edward Amory Winslow titled his 1943 history of public health *The Conquest of Epidemic Disease*, he was referring to the implementation of programs to defeat the spread of germs. When U.S. newspapers trumpeted "victory" over polio in 1955, they referred to the nationwide immunization program (the 1954 field trial of the new vaccine involved 1,830,000 children in forty-four states) and to the specific germ, poliovirus. But by the 1970s, it was possible to attribute an epidemic to virtually any cause that could be delivered plausibly to a public that was awaiting reassuring news of the cause of epidemic illness—wanting to know who the enemy was and what army was going to stop it. The rise in syphilis in the '70s was caused by the popularity of the birth-control pill or by promiscuity or homosexuality, it would be said, but the mysterious drama of human sexual relations would not have to play a part in the causal story. The swine flu affair of 1976 was called a fiasco not because influenza viruses' interactions with human and animal populations are complex but because the weapons simply misfired, or the enemy, H1N1 flu virus, failed to appear for battle. Very simple stories would account for the epidemics and near-epidemics that captured fearful fantasies of the destabilization of modern life.

With modern technology, the ability to isolate specific causes for diseases of public-health importance, and the capacity to delude ourselves that illness could be conquered, medical scientists and public-health officials would eventually declare victory over all of the traditional forms of contagion that vexed modern society, like VD. The new scientific machinery of health improvement seemed capable of convincing people that science was invincible and epidemics could be stopped.

CHAPTER 6

POSTMODERN EPIDEMICS

Whenever an evil chance event—a sudden storm or a
crop failure or a plague—strikes a community, the suspicion is aroused that custom has been offended in
some way or that new practices have to be devised to
propitiate a new demonic power and caprice.

—Friedrich Nietzsche, Daybreak

In the late 1970s, the understanding of epidemics began to shift.
That epidemic illness resulted from discrete and identifiable causes
remained unassailable, but the capacity of medical science to provide
relief from some epidemic threats, like VD and polio, stoked a hunger
for preventing all of them—and a corresponding surprise when it
turned out that epidemics might strike anyway. In the developed world
the rapid pace of technological advance provoked new anxieties about
modern life, particularly worries about dangers that might be lurking
inside the very technology that made life safer and more secure.

With increasingly influential news media often bent on arousing
those same new fears as a way of selling newspapers or TV advertising
time, the demand for protection from alleged dangers no longer came
from individuals' personal sense of dread alone or from powerful
groups pushing an agenda. By the '70s, the clamor to identify threats

and prevent epidemics was so powerfully provoked by media reports that when the media were silent it could seem that the entire society was complacent. Continuing fears that sexual misbehavior could destabilize society came to the fore in the context of anxieties about modernity, expressed as suspicions that new products or practices harbored threats. In the past, people had understood epidemic threats by applying fears internal to the social psyche to outside causes, creating hysterias about foreign perfidy, portraying immigration as social pollution, or suppressing the genetically "unwholesome." The new epidemic thinking involved fears that were increasingly provided externally by the media. At the same time, the alleged source of threats turned from outside to inside. Increasingly, danger was said to begin with intimate decision making and the use of new products.

In 1978, a Colorado physician described severe shock in seven children, ages eight to eighteen, hypothesizing that a toxin elaborated by a strain of *Staphylococcus aureus* bacteria was responsible. The following year three similar cases appeared among Wisconsin women. By May 1980, fifty-five cases had been reported, and the CDC asserted that toxic shock syndrome seemed to be associated with menstruation, specifically with tampons—bringing TSS to the nation's attention as an epidemic linked to women of reproductive age. Later that year, officials reported a statistical association between TSS and the use of Rely brand "superabsorbent" tampons. Procter & Gamble, the manufacturer of the Rely brand, withdrew the product from the market and mounted the most expensive advertising campaign ever intended to discourage a product's use. There was no evidence that Rely was causing TSS—the advertising campaign was a transparent effort to repair P&G's possibly compromised public image as well as to avoid liability. But it contributed to the understanding of TSS as a pathology that symbolized a problem with female fertility.

The TSS epidemic was a media-driven health crisis. Toxic shock syndrome isn't contagious, but it was discussed as though it were. The scare aimed at women of reproductive age was created by media responding to government reports—which were themselves influenced by media attention. Although TSS is evidently associated with bacterial infection, it was never very common, even among young women; it was never restricted to women (14 of the first 408 cases of severe TSS were in men); and no unique causative role of tampons was ever established. Articles in the popular press about TSS in the early 1980s almost always focused on the most severe cases. And even after stories appeared describing TSS among men and children, the ill were almost always defined as menstruating females. Journalists being particularly receptive to the story of mishap in association with menstruation, they dramatized the TSS epidemic as a supposed dysfunction in female genital habits. Into the 1980s, the sexual female remained both vulnerable and dangerous.

The TSS story, as told in the media and by complaisant officials, was a new take on the old story that modern sexual arrangements invite danger and that defiance of nature with technological innovation tempts fate. There was the "superabsorbent" tampon, the device that might serve a woman's attempt to confound nature's bloodiness with a new industrial product. There was the special risk to "women of childbearing age," the phrase itself implying that a woman able to have children might *not* have children and might even continue to have sexual intercourse without plans for propagating the race or forming a family, and further implying that as sexual relations had become playthings, fertility had become irrelevant.

The turn in epidemic thought was even more evident when an outbreak of respiratory illness, with 128 cases and 29 deaths, occurred among the middle-aged and older men attending an American Legion convention in Philadelphia in July 1976. Legionnaires' disease became a news-making medical mystery by early that fall. When the cause of the outbreak, a tiny bacterium, was isolated in early 1977, it was found to be capable of living in the moist climate of air-conditioning systems. By 1978, similar outbreaks had been identified and attributed to the bacterium *Legionella pneumophila.* Legionnaires' disease came to be seen as a kind of caution about the potentially nasty consequences of modern life. As one writer put it,

"A new human disease had emerged in 1976, brought from ancient obscurity by the modern invention of air conditioning."

Legionnaires' wasn't really new in 1976, though. The facts had been bent, or simply ignored, to accommodate a narrative in which a dangerous new threat multiplying silently deep inside a modern convenience emerges unheralded. In truth, once *L. pneumophila* had been identified, a look at records showed that the very same organism had been isolated in cases going back to 1947. Outbreaks had taken place as early as 1957. *Legionella pneumophila* hadn't "emerged" from hiding (although it had indeed become more common in the '70s). And legionellosis didn't depend on air-conditioning: outbreaks can occur in association with any sort of stored water supply. But the full truth isn't always important. The smaller facts—the middle-aged men, the "new" disease, and the air-conditioning—fit better to the story, the metaphor of danger lurking inside the technology that makes us comfortable. Legionnaires' became an "emergence," an example of the supposed stealth of germ agents and hidden dangers of contemporary life.

In viewing Legionnaires' disease as an epidemic crisis, the outward view with which people had always looked at epidemic threats turned inward. If American Legion members, middle-aged or older white men—people bearing the marks of privilege in American society, that is—could be sickened by a new disease, an infection that had suddenly "emerged" from air-conditioning ducts in a hotel, then anyone might be at risk. It wasn't just the outsider who could be suspect. The threat might come from within the culture. What could be more quintessentially American than air-conditioning in a hotel in Philadelphia?

Like TSS, Legionnaires' disease revealed a shift in American fears and a concomitant change in how people weighed risks. The germ of the new epidemic might be anywhere. If the danger of infection could be anywhere, then it was incumbent on us to look even more deeply to find out who was likely to be susceptible and who not. The new thinking meant that people must try to discern the carrier state lurking behind the healthy exterior. With the birth of emerging threats, we turned the disease-dreading gaze inward toward ourselves and our society.

To locate the origin of the epidemic deep within society or self is to make ambiguous what had once been clear. Labeling an already-scorned group as the carriers of disease, as Irish immigrants were held accountable for cholera, was once a simple anathema. In the new epidemic, to be characterized as a risk group would denote a lack of political worth. Disease could be claimed, embraced as an emblem of identity, or redefined as a violation of civil rights, even as it continued to be wielded as a weapon to discredit the unwanted.

The shift was subtle at first, in the '70s. But it hinted at a revision of the picture of the epidemic just in time for the arrival of the era's greatest disease event.

AN EXTRAORDINARY EPIDEMIC

It was almost certainly in New York that the AIDS virus made its American landfall, sometime in the 1970s. By the time AIDS was recognized officially, in a June 1981 publication by the Centers for Disease Control (although it was not yet called AIDS), the gay press in New York was already speculating about a rumored new "gay cancer."

In May 1981 the *New York Native*, a leading gay newspaper, published an article by Dr. Harold Ross titled "Playing It Safe." In it, Ross noted that genital infections seemed to be on the increase among young gay men who were having sex with many other men. "Everyone has a friend," he wrote, "who has a friend who has just contracted hepatitis or amebas or venereal warts or herpes or whatever for the umpteenth time." Ross could not have known that CDC officials were already investigating what they thought was a new disease that was, somehow, associated with homosexual intercourse.

In the first few weeks of 1981, the CDC's Epidemic Intelligence Service officer in Los Angeles was informed of some mysterious cases of infections and a rare cancer called Kaposi's sarcoma occurring in people with immune dysregulation. In New York, two physicians investigating genital and anal herpes among gay men, and canvassing other physicians with gay patients to assemble a case series, were in touch with the sexually transmitted diseases branch of the CDC. By late spring of 1981, James Curran and Harold Jaffe of the CDC were beginning to investigate their hunch that something about male-male sex was linked to a new outbreak. As cases were being reported in sexually active gay men, investigators presumed it was caused by a transmissible pathogen, and they fixed on a virus. Investigations the CDC had been conducting in the late 1970s into hepatitis B and gonorrhea transmission among gay men segued into research on the new disease.

It was a foregone conclusion that the new contagion was associated with homosexual activity—either because gay men were acquiring new sex partners at high rates or because of some particular male-male sex practice. We now know that what the CDC investigators were studying, in New York, Los Angeles, and San Francisco, was not unique to homosexual men, even in 1981. Curran and Jaffe were not wrong: a new agent was indeed spreading among highly sexually active men in America's cities. But it would take years for investigators to amass the evidence needed to inform carefully drawn hypotheses about cause. For many observers, foregone conclusions were easier.

The CDC's suspicion that a new form of gay-related contagion was afoot was not communicated widely in 1981. Although the Epidemic Intelligence Service officer in Los Angeles was aware of it, the epidemiologist in the San Francisco health department was not. Gay activists and, in particular, the gay press were kept out of the picture—perhaps for reasons of tact, as the CDC is an agency of a national government that was not then inclined to recognize the gay movement, or simply because the investigators felt their theories were too speculative to be shared publicly. In an interview with New York City's Epidemic Intelligence Service officer in late May 1981, Dr. Larry Mass, a reporter for the *New York Native*, learned that eleven cases of unexplained pneumonia had appeared in the city's hospitals in just the past four months; the pneumonia was caused by *Pneumocystis carinii*, an organism that generally produces disease only among people with compromised immune systems. The EIS officer told Mass that four of the five individuals hospitalized at Bellevue Hospital with this pneumonia were gay men. But, the officer said, rumors of a new "gay" disease were "for the most part unfounded." Thus it came as a surprise to some when the CDC published the first report on five cases of pneumocystis pneumonia, all gay men, in early June. It was the first official notice of what we now call AIDS.

Almost immediately, the new disease became turf in the battleground for gay identity. Epidemics, as this one of a yet-unnamed disease revealed, would continue to serve to distance a group from the rest of society, but might also consolidate a group's identity. The epidemic would bring into sharp focus the new tendency to see disease threats as coming from fissures within our own society.

Shortly after the first report of the new disease, a CDC official told *The Advocate*, an L.A.-based gay newspaper, that immune impairment, not homosexuality, was responsible for the new pneumonia cases. But a second article in an official CDC publication, which appeared on July 4, 1981, explicitly mentioned homosexuality as a characteristic of new cases (although it was cautious about any implications as to cause). Mass, writing in the *New York Native* in late July 1981 after talking to physicians in New York, cognizant now of a potential connection between the new condition and homosexual intercourse, found the "most immediately seductive environmental explanation" to be that the new disease was "being caused by an infectious or otherwise cancerous agent." In late May 1982, Mass reported that there was no evidence that the new disease was caused by a contagious agent. Frequent intercourse with a variety of partners, though, might be, as he put it, a "risk factor."

By the time the new disease was named AIDS, in the summer of 1982, ambivalence infused the conversation. In a society that was still uncomfortable about public discussions of male-male sex and deeply bigoted about homosexuality, to speak about AIDS at all was to risk being "outed" as gay or, for a heterosexual, being misidentified as gay.

The CDC had received reports of 593 individuals with AIDS between June 1981 and mid-September 1982, and 75 percent of the cases were listed as "homosexual or bisexual men." More than 40 percent of those men were already dead by the end of the summer of 1982. An outbreak of a horrifying new disease that was linked to gay sexual practice and thus might somehow be "gay" in its essence, as TB was once thought to be artistic, and later Jewish, and as polio was thought to be Italian, presented the intriguing possibility that gayness might be consolidated in what Susan Sontag called a homosexual ethnicity—a nationhood "whose distinctive folkloric custom was sexual voracity." But some gay men were increasingly suspicious of the identification of AIDS as a gay disease. Perhaps these suspicions were amplified by the presumption that all gay men were sexually insatiable, so far from the truth. It would have been easy, especially for men whose sex lives were relatively sedate, to wonder if the allegations that AIDS was associated with homosexuality were merely a new example of the traditional gesture, blaming contagion on an unwanted group. Many publications proffered apocalyptic scenarios that fixed not on sexual transmission of a germ but on homosexuality per se as the cause of a coming disaster. The *Toronto Star*, London's *Sun*, *Newsweek*, and a number of other newspapers wrote of a gay or homosexual "plague."

AIDS, and eventually the concept of the epidemic writ large in the modern era, would become about who we are and what we do more than it was about the epidemic's source. Implicitly signaling the new story, the CDC wrote in its official report in September 1982 that AIDS could be read in terms of risk groups. These groups included: "Homosexual or bisexual males—75%, intravenous drug abusers with no history of homosexual activity—13%, Haitians with neither a history of homosexuality or intravenous drug abuse—6%, persons with hemophilia A with no other risk factors—0.3%, and persons in none of the other groups—5%." AIDS, the federal agency was telling us, would not follow the rhetorical tropes that had been standard, neither the germ-laden narrative of perilous foreigners nor the facile suspicion of loose women. AIDS would not follow the path of cholera, polio, and TB in being ascribed to immigrants alone. It would not be seen simply as a retribution for sexual license (although many commentators would want it to seem so). It would become entangled with race—but in a way far more complex than the simplistic notions of the Nazis or the eugenicists would have allowed. AIDS would not be ordinary.

Would the CDC wholeheartedly embrace a sub-rosa campaign to depict the new disease as an extraordinary and entirely new sort of visitation? Was it part of an effort by a socially conservative government (Ronald Reagan had taken office in 1981) to marginalize gay men and drug addicts? Was it an attempt to play up to heterosexual fears that homosexuality was disrupting the social fabric? An article in the *Village Voice* transmitted gay men's suspicion that the government was at least indifferent to what some believed to be unique suffering, objecting to the "plague of medical jargon." In "1,112 and Counting," which appeared in the *Native* in March 1983, the playwright and activist Larry Kramer charged the CDC with ineffectual surveillance, the U.S. National Institutes of Health (the main federal health-research agency) with inadequate investigation of AIDS, the *New York Times* with inadequate coverage, and New York's mayor, Edward Koch, with insouciance. And he ended with a call for civil disobedience. Kramer's piece was a nonviolent call to arms, a swipe of the glove. For proponents of gay identity, the duel was on. Government officials would be the opponent.

But there probably was no concerted effort on the part of government officials to withhold information from gay men. In a January 1982 article, CDC investigator James Curran wrote that his organization was gathering data to "identify risk if not causative factors." The

CDC epidemiologists were interested in the cause of the new disease, believed it to be a virus, and suspected that something about gay sex figured in its etiology—rectal bleeding, drugs like amyl nitrite used to enhance orgasm, or another factor. Whatever the officials believed, they couched their statements only in the language of risk.

Risk, the epidemiologist's probability statement, became linked to and in some ways substituted for cause. "Risk" sounds like the crapshoot of everyday life. "Cause" is an allegation that has moral resonances, useful in the political debates over sexual tolerance and civil rights. Translating observations about risk into presumptions of cause was not the work of health officials. In fact, the CDC investigators spoke of risk because they weren't sure of the cause. It was a variegated mix of gay activists, politicians promoting "family values," advocates of "social justice," pundits wielding weapons of the culture wars, and journalists looking for a story who began to talk about male-male sex and heroin injection as causes of AIDS.

DEBATES ABOUT DEVIANCE

The translation from risk statement to causal claim proceeded in two stages. First there was an argument about sexual license—an old debate, but in the AIDS context one that was no longer framed in the grammar of marriage, fidelity, and male-female differences. Now the question about the acceptability of sexual license became an inquiry into the nature of male sexual need. Fears of homosexuality and, for some homosexual men, fears that their hard-won identity would be suppressed by the heterosexual culture, drove the debate. Next came a clear-cut debate over private individuals' public obligations. The pressing question was whether the social compact demanded that everyone comply with the larger society's needs or moral expectations—even in the most private of realms, the bedroom.

By the middle of 1982, the most vocal gay men had taken sides: one group, calling itself "sex-positive," held that multifarious sexual liaisons were so intrinsic to the newly consolidated gay identity that they should not be forgone even in the face of a frightening disease. The other contended that, as Dr. Joseph Sonnabend put it in a September 1982 *New York Native* article, "promiscuity is bad for your health." In November of that year, "Two Men Declare War on Promiscuity," another opinion piece in the *Native*, called sexual excess the cause of AIDS. By April 1983, a newly formed group of gay physicians, the American Association of Physicians for Human Rights, recommended that gay men reduce their number of sexual partners, especially men who themselves had had many different partners. *The Advocate* countered that the "AIDS crisis has given [promiscuity] a deadly cast just as it was about to shake off its old moral associations."

AIDS was never strictly a homosexual disease or even purely a sexually transmitted disease. The AIDS virus is spread far more effectively when the blood of an infected person is inoculated into an uninfected one—as happens with transfusions and the transfer of blood products such as clotting factor for hemophiliacs, and with the reuse of medical injection equipment.* Anal sexual contact is slightly more effective at moving the virus from person to person than is penile-vaginal sex, but transmission through contaminated intravenous needles, or by transfusing contaminated blood itself, has generally been responsible when there has been a rapid amplification of a geographically limited focus of infection. That is what happened in the United States, where initial infection occurred in the '70s among drug injectors in New York City and quickly spread.

Because sexual intercourse is much more common than transfusions or intravenous injections, sexual spread allows viral infection to expand effectively, if slowly, through the population. Sexual transmission of the AIDS virus has been responsible for a high prevalence of

---

*Both improper sterilization in medical facilities and reuse of contaminated needles and syringes by injectors of illicit drugs have been involved in the spread of the virus by this route.

infections in some places, especially where the practice of concurrent partnerships is common (parts of Africa, for instance). Where many people have long-term, concurrent sexual contact with a few partners each, a high prevalence of AIDS-virus infection can result even though nobody in the society has a very high number of sexual partners in his or her lifetime. But in societies where so-called serial monogamy is the norm, sexual transmission is inefficient for creating an epidemic. Transmission of the virus via intercourse is inherently of low probability and people who do contract the virus are highly infectious to others only for a relatively short period (usually a few weeks; after that, they are less likely to transmit the virus, infectious but at a lesser level). Therefore, incipient outbreaks of AIDS virus infection don't usually extend to the larger population suddenly and dramatically because of sexual contact.*

The popular discussion of AIDS at the time it entered the world stage was not centered on the facts of transmission, though. In the United States, anxiety over sexual "deviance" or simple discomfiture over sex made it important for some to indict homosexuality as the hidden fertilizer that would make American soil friendlier to the growth of the epidemic. Officials and corporate media colluded, albeit not by outright agreement: they fixed homosexuality, now tainted with AIDS, as a vein that might run through all sexual events. There was, for instance, the pronouncement by U.S. Secretary of Health and Human Services Dr. Otis Bowen that "when a person has sex, they're not just having it with that partner, they're having it with everybody that partner had it with for the past 10 years." Why create such a virtual chain of sexual liaisons except to imply that even heterosexual coition is just one remove from same-sex intercourse—dangerous no matter how careful one might be in

---

*One exception was created by the sexual practices of some gay men in the 1970s who had a great many partners. That would have allowed for rapid spread of viral infection through sex alone.

choosing a partner? Even Bowen, who seemed to have little investment in proving that AIDS was America's punishment for tolerating homosexuals, couldn't quite manage a metaphor for epidemic
peril that did not imply homosexual hazard. Sex itself made sexual
license tantamount to a germ by the 1980s.

The debate about sexual license in the abstract coalesced around
a discussion of bathhouses and bars where men could meet other
men for sex. Some observers estimated that 15,000 men visited the
baths in San Francisco every weekend in the '70s. There might have
been an even larger crowd in New York. By 1980 one infectious-
disease doctor said that it wasn't unusual to find men who had sex
with more than 500 other men in the course of a year. The multiplicity of contacts in the bars and baths would have made them
ideal for spreading any sexually transmissible pathogen—even the
AIDS virus, with a relatively low probability of transmission per
contact, will spread efficiently if there are a great many contacts in a
short period of time.

In late 1982, Joseph Sonnabend, the New York physician who
wrote the "promiscuity" article, suggested closing the bars and baths.
His article in a professional journal on the possible causes of AIDS
drew attention to the role of multiple sexual exposures. Larry Mass,
the physician-reporter for the Native, responded that closing the bars
and baths would be hasty and would cause people "to blame the [gay]
community [which] is not the cause . . . but the victim of AIDS." By
March 1984, a respected gay physician told Randy Shilts, writing for
the San Francisco Chronicle, that a gay man newly arrived in San
Francisco would be well advised "not to have sex in the traditional
sense of the word." Closing the businesses that promoted what he
called high-risk sex would set a model for the nation and help reduce
the spread of AIDS, the physician claimed.

In 1983, the health commissioner for the city of San Francisco
moved to close six baths, four gay sex clubs, two movie theaters, and
two gay bookstores, despite objections from a CDC sociologist, an

epidemiologist with the New York City Health Department, and others who insisted that closure would have no effect on the growth of the AIDS epidemic. Some gay activists, including Shilts, supported the move. So did many in the city's government, who had to allay fears that homosexual activity was endangering the entire population. Others, including Mass, were opposed. In the end, the effort was foiled by a restraining order issued by California state court justice Roy Wonder in November 1984. New York State moved against baths and bars in New York City, despite the New York City Health Department's objection, padlocking the notorious Mine Shaft, a club on Manhattan's West Side, on November 7, 1985.*

In practical terms, not much ever came of the argument over closing the baths. But the debate reframed the AIDS epidemic, displacing it from the themes of earlier ones. The concept of the epidemic as punishment for failures of probity and/or piety (and as offering the opportunity for redemption from them), so common during the nineteenth and early twentieth centuries, faded as AIDS spread. Only those who rejected categorically the notion that homosexuality might account for any recognizable part of American private life—people like evangelist Jerry Falwell, who called homosexuality a "perverted lifestyle"**—persisted in viewing AIDS as a result of impiety. Referring to bathhouse sex as "sub-animal behavior," Falwell asserted that "when you violate moral, health, and hygiene laws you reap the whirlwind."

More generally, the new epidemic was defined in terms of prudence, the limits of privacy, and the reach of social obligations. AIDS

---

*Remarkably, the Mine Shaft was the only establishment catering to a homosexual clientele ever shuttered by the 1985 official order. Eager to convey the impression that its concern about the transmission of genital diseases was not discriminatory against gays, New York State also acted against Plato's Retreat, a heterosexual swingers' club.

**Falwell made this remark in a televised conversation on AIDS in the summer of 1983.

was said to have "targeted" gays—was said to be, in Larry Kramer's word, a gay "holocaust." Kramer both identified the gay man in America's contemporary gaze with the Jew in that of the Nazis and redefined AIDS as a massacre. From this perspective, AIDS contributed to the victimization of what had become, as a pointed reaction to the heterosexual-companionate-marriage norm of modern industrial society, a quasi-ethnic grouping, a gay tribe. From the other direction, Patrick Buchanan spoke for those who feared or despised sexual transgression when he described AIDS as evidence that gayness equals death. "It has long been the defiant slogan of the gay rights movement that, so long as we don't injure anyone, what we do is our own business," Buchanan wrote. "If promiscuous homosexuals in the urban centers of New York and San Francisco are capable of transmitting death with a casual sexual contact, their slogan, to put it mildly, would no longer seem to apply." Laden with valences of exclusion, purposive abandonment, and sexual misalliance, AIDS roiled the American medical and social scenes.

Understood as a kind of opportunism on nature's part that took advantage of failures of prudence, AIDS came to be defined as a crisis not of invasion or pollution but of identity and "lifestyles." AIDS, with the new inward-focused fear, came to be seen as a crisis involving the so-called stigmatization of certain lifestyles and the denial of equal opportunity (opportunity being understood as the wherewithal to follow the "chosen lifestyle"). The epidemic came to represent a failure not of capital but of will. It seemed to be not a disaster that befalls the destitute, as Virchow had seen typhus a century and a half before, but rather the result of a lack of so-called social capital, a paucity of civic engagement or trust, a failure of the system to accommodate everyone, or a failure of everyone to get with the program. AIDS encapsulated anxieties about modern life, the imperative to be productive, the importance of belonging to the right group, and the will to succeed.

The bathhouse controversy enacted an ancient drama featuring freedom and responsibility. The gay men who argued for padlocking the baths wanted the authorities to use the might of the state to protect the weak against the licentious. It would have made little difference to the continuance of the epidemic—by the time the controversy broke, the virus had already expanded dramatically through the population of highly sexually active gay men. But it might have made a small difference in practical terms and would have had tremendous symbolic value. Specifically, the pro-closure forces thought the state must help those men who could not resist the allure of the sexual carnival in the baths and bars, or who did not know that disease could be spread there, to protect themselves from themselves. They wanted officials to ensure the safety not only of behaviors that are accepted practice, like automobile driving, but of those activities deemed transgressive by most Americans, including male-male sex. Michael Callen, founder of the People With AIDS Coalition, explained that "the logic behind temporary closure of commercial sex establishments is not to make it impossible for gay men to engage in high-risk behavior—but to make it much more difficult." Sexual liberty that activists like Callen envisioned was to be made real by limiting it when necessary. Just as we know that there is free speech in part because we acknowledge that we are *not* free to harm people with deliberate lies (yelling "fire" in the proverbial crowded theater), the full realization of sexual freedom would require limits on sexual expression.

Officials genuinely did not want to supervise sexual behavior, even if the law permitted them to do so (anti-sodomy laws were still on some states' statute books in that day, and would be upheld in the Supreme Court's 1986 *Bowers v. Hardwick* decision). As late as 1995, even with some gay activists arguing that a "moderate restriction in civil liberties," as one put it, was acceptable if it would help gay men to avoid further spread of AIDS, officials in New York City closed just two gay theaters and one sex club, apparently hoping to settle the argument about the permissibility of sex in an outbreak without making any grand gestures. The controversy among gay men about what should be permissible sexually in a disease outbreak surely stayed the creation of official policy.

Many commentators, including but not limited to gay activists, joined Larry Kramer in interpreting the absence of policy on male-male sex as a sign of government indifference. Others went further, finding the very framing of the AIDS discussion around homosexuality to be a disappointing expression of America's disgust for male-male sex, or for sex in general. Thomas Stoddard of the New York Civil Liberties Union felt that "homophobes" might make use of bathhouse closure to press an illiberal agenda—and that officials who would normally be respectful of liberty might be drawn along by the rationale of protecting the public's health. "If bathhouses, why not movie houses," Stoddard asked, "and if movie houses, why not gay bars, and if we close all those dangerous places, why not criminalize the underlying conduct?" By 1985, it was barely possible to talk about AIDS without mentioning homosexuality, to talk about the gay-rights movement without mentioning AIDS, or to think about civil rights without invoking both sexual liberty and the AIDS epidemic.

No longer aimed at germ-carrying foreigners, with AIDS the epidemic story became part of the circumscribing of a native and largely white group of gay men. When syphilis accusations were leveled at black men in the South in the 1930s, when San Francisco's Chinese were held responsible for spreading plague in 1900, and when the Irish were targeted during the cholera outbreak of 1849, campaigns for civil rights were in part a demand that the victims not be blamed for the illness in question. With AIDS in the mid-'80s, the campaign for civil rights trod a trickier path: gay activists had to reject any automatic association of AIDS with homosexuality so as to argue that gays' rights were violated when, for instance, there were calls to bar homosexuals from school teaching. But activists also had to acknowledge the association of gayness with AIDS in order to agitate for more research and treatment. With some gay men declaring a paradoxical ownership over the ghastly mortal toll of AIDS, with both activists and public-health professionals split over the advisability of state control of sex establishments like the baths (a divide that seemed to stand for disagreement over whether to approve or abhor sexual abandon), and with many voices demanding that federal agencies give AIDS more attention and funding, the public discussion about AIDS became the leading example of the new, inward-looking nature of the epidemic.

THE MIXING OF CAUSE AND EFFECT

In the internalized epidemic, the name of a threat has to tell us something about what we suspect we harbor within us. When the CDC coined the name for the new disease during the summer of 1982, acquired immune deficiency syndrome sounded both important and vague; the word "syndrome," which had typically denoted a medical mystery, seemed apt. Paradoxically, although the disease was already dreadful to the few people who knew about it by mid-1982, it came to be called by the acronym that, to most people, still sounded innocent: AIDS.

Officials modified the name to HIV/AIDS in the late 1980s. HIV/AIDS, which quickly became de rigueur, made the point that we had moved past the fixations of modernism and into new territory. By blotting out the distinction between cause and effect, HIV/AIDS made infection itself the illness.

Until at least the mid-twentieth century, the simple causal narrative of germs and disease allowed people to suspect the poor or the foreign. But AIDS exploded the myth of the conquest of contagion and seemed to invalidate that simple causal (germ) story on which the conquest myth was based. HIV/AIDS could not be comprehended by attending only to infection and the virus's ostensible effect. Implicitly, we would fail to recognize the unprecedented nature of this disease were we to name it after the causative virus alone (HIV disease, say), and we would fail to recognize the true inner source of its emergence were we to call it the old-fashioned acquired immune deficiency syndrome. Withdrawing from the world of observables and implying that what is inside (an infection, imprudence, impiety, or immorality) is the same as what is outside (a disease), "HIV/AIDS" effectively illustrated a new epidemic narrative wherein there were threats emerging from so deep within individual psyches or society's soul that the cause could not be identified except by referring to the outcome. If you had the disease, you had whatever caused it.

After AIDS had been around for a decade, it seemed as if the simple certainties of germ theory and the hopes of eugenic theory had been repackaged, with the putative cause no longer an invisible germ but an invisible behavior—unprotected sex. Society's dread of instability was remade. We ourselves were the threat.

THE BEHAVIORAL TURN: EDUCATION AS POLICY

Gay activists were wrong to see the U.S. federal government as entirely inactive on AIDS. On the contrary, AIDS was the subject of considerable activity at many levels of government—but the activity was toward shutting out any understanding of AIDS other than as a matter of behavioral excess. AIDS quickly became a *behavioral epidemic*.

That health professionals in the United States had to fight in order to do nothing more in response to AIDS than proscribe sex with "multiple partners" or promote the use of latex condoms shows how hard it was for Americans to see AIDS as anything other than an outbreak of bad behavior. Although a blood test for exposure to the AIDS virus went into use for screening blood donations in late 1984 and became commercially available in 1985, there was no policy on testing for the virus until 1987, when the definition of AIDS expanded to include diagnosis by blood test of HIV infection. Needle- and syringe-exchange programs (in which drug users are given sterile injection equipment when they turn in used equipment) were known to be effective at interrupting transmission of the AIDS virus, but such exchange schemes were implemented only slowly in the United States. As late as 2008, a prohibition on exchange programs in the city of Washington, D.C., was lifted only as part of omnibus spending legislation, and the president immediately sought to reinstate the ban.

But virtually all constituencies could agree to see AIDS as a matter of behavior. As John-Manuel Andriote recounts in *Victory Deferred*, his masterful history of AIDS in relation to the gay movement, many gay men felt they had to dispel the opprobrium of American society by making sex safer. To accomplish safer sex required touting the condom.

The old truth that each disease is caused by its own germ had always been too simple to describe an epidemic both fully and validly, and with AIDS it came at last into question. Indeed, whether HIV was a necessary cause of AIDS became a topic of some controversy. But when the adequacy of the germ explanation gave way, it did not spur a richer and truer understanding. We did not replace germ theory with a sense that epidemic disease arises when a complex of social factors conjoin and a germ opportunistically enters the group of people caught by those complications (although some who studied AIDS did their best to popularize this view). We began to speak as if we were skeptical that there could be any tangible cause of an epidemic at all. Instead of causes we spoke of risks, and when we spoke of risks we often meant something very vague—an amorphous combination of vulnerability, poor self-esteem, and imprudent behavior.

As the AIDS toll mounted, health officials, gay leaders, academics, the media, and essentially everyone else who was involved in the AIDS world entered the agreement that behavior was the key to AIDS—key to causing it, understanding it, and controlling it. Gay activists and liberal health professionals created an unlikely alliance with the evangelists (like Falwell) and the social conservatives (like Buchanan), who saw homosexual behavior as a threat. The health officials and gay leaders thought behavior was important to social wel-

fare. The evangelists and conservatives thought behavior was important to public morality. As early as 1986, the report of a meeting of
AIDS scientists at the Coolfont Center in West Virginia emphasized
that information and educational campaigns were essential to AIDS
prevention. A report by the National Academy of Science's Institute
of Medicine that same year found that AIDS education in the United
States was "woefully inadequate." The Surgeon General's first report
on AIDS, also issued in 1986, advocated "frank, open discussions on
AIDS" between parents and children. Early in 1987, the British government sent a pamphlet to every household that read, "AIDS. Don't
die of ignorance." With information about behavior at the center of
the new epidemic, everybody could be on equal footing in our distress.

The epidemiologists' statement of risk pertains exclusively to
groups, a claim about the relatively high probability of an event
(AIDS, in this case) occurring within the group compared with the
probability among the public at large. The statement about risk behavior signaled a shift from describing epidemics in terms of groups
to blaming them on our, or someone's, behavior. Risky behavior was
said to be the cause of AIDS, therefore, with "risky" standing for almost anything that could have to do with sex and, usually, what the
speaker's or writer's audience would find distasteful. The 1982–1983
list of risk groups was revised over time, and by the late '80s it had become a list of risk behaviors. The list included intravenous drug use
and unprotected sex (it continues to include them today), but being
Haitian was dropped. The turn from risk group to risk behavior was a
sign of an important change in thinking, a behavioral turn, wherein
behavior as risk became behavior as cause. By the '90s, acts that
might lead the person performing them to become "risky," such as
excessive drinking, became relevant to the hazy but overheated discussion of "causes of HIV/AIDS." Even states of mind (despair,
"AIDS fatigue") became relevant once the behavioral turn had been
introduced. The cause of AIDS moved ever further within the individual and, implicitly, within society.

With this behavioral turn, a new moralism insisted on mores of sexual propriety—updated for the AIDS era but no less stridently upheld than they had been in the Progressive movement at the turn of the century. In American culture, unprotected sex came to be discussed in pitying or disapproving tones, sometimes seeming tantamount to sin. If the AIDS discussion abandoned old assumptions about germs and tensions about wealth, it acquired equally powerful new ones about prudence, opportunity, and social compact.

Condoms came out of the closet. By 1988, Surgeon General C. Everett Koop was able to mail to every household in America a pamphlet advising that a condom be used for intercourse if it was impossible to be in a mutually monogamous relationship. There was debate over whether and how condoms could be advertised on television. The archdiocese of New York opposed a plan to make condoms available in New York City's public schools, leading to cessation of the program. The activist organization ACT UP retaliated by staging a die-in at St. Patrick's Cathedral in New York City in 1989, in part to dramatize the conflict between the church's moral stance about the unnaturalness of homosexuality and its belief in the sanctity of life but also, pointedly, to direct attention to the church's refusal to endorse condom campaigns.

In the behavioral turn, everyone would agree to revile sexual transgression. The old disapproval of the sexually licentious, once couched in terms of religious impiety, came back in the new terms of imprudence about health. There were differences in the definition of transgression, to be sure. Most health professionals saw no particular threat in same-sex intercourse per se, only in the way and frequency with which it was conducted. The other school saw a deep moral threat in male-male intercourse, at whatever frequency. But those lines blurred and changed over time. The centerpiece of the agreement was that the public's health depended on adjusting behavior to conform sexually. AIDS policy would become little more than delivering reminders about how that conformity should be accomplished.

It would come to be called "health education" or, in a reminder about the new elusiveness of cause, "risk-reduction education." But it would be, in essence, no different from the sexual messages of the preceding centuries: sexual misadventure leads to ruin.

Educating people about healthful habits had been a part of the American public health movement since the early 1900s. But before the advent of AIDS, never had the entirety of disease-prevention policy been to tell people what they should stop doing. Even the high moralism of VD control in the Progressive era advocated Wasserman testing and control of prostitution as well as reform of sexual habits. In the AIDS era, behavior control *was* disease control.

EDUCATION IN LIEU OF POLICY

The condom became the iconic assertion of the impending "conquest" of AIDS—not the way vaccination supposedly had conquered germs in the twentieth century but through education about avoiding risk. The altar of safe sex was one at which everyone could worship— gay liberationists, health officials, and politicians alike. The condom became a symbol of safe sex to those who wanted to preserve liberties around sexual choice.

Debate did continue over what form the education about sex and AIDS should take—should it be abstinence until and outside marriage, should it be so-called partner reduction, should it be condom promotion? But that was a shell game. What role parents and other nonprofessionals should take in setting education policy is an important question, reflected in the debate over AIDS prevention education. But there was no important public-health question at stake. By the late 1980s and early '90s, in the United States and Western Europe, the AIDS virus was moving indolently through sexual contact. In those circumstances, the exact mode by which prevention of sexual spread was implemented would have made little difference to the overall level of infection in the population. Reducing the rate at which new sex partners are acquired, increasing condom use, delaying sexual debut, increasing monogamy, or any combination thereof might have made a small difference if everyone adopted the recommended behavior. But with sexual spread of virus a low-frequency event, no intervention could have made a big difference at the population level.*

What would have made a big difference to the AIDS epidemic remained unspoken. The AIDS virus passes efficiently from person to person in blood transfusions. Considerable outcry over the safety of the blood supply arose in the early 1980s, after a report of the death of a twenty-month-old child made clear the potential for AIDS transmission by transfusion. Scandals in which the virus was disseminated because of poor policing of blood supplies later contributed to the outcry. News of an event in France broke in 1991 and enjoyed high-profile media coverage as it made its way through the courts. The discovery in 1992 that tennis star Arthur Ashe had been infected by a blood transfusion about ten years earlier (Ashe died of AIDS in February 1993) was also part of the furor over blood safety. Yet the connection between AIDS and blood had little impact on the centrality of sex in the public discussion of AIDS. And the blood-blood spread of the AIDS virus that occurs because of the sharing of equipment used for self-injection by users of illicit drugs (heroin and cocaine, predominantly) hardly entered the conversation.

Rarely did anyone speak of AIDS as a blood-borne illness. Instead, there were controversies over the blood-banking business, nominally

---

*Condoms are very effective at preventing transmission of the AIDS virus during intercourse, if one partner is infected and the other is not. Recommending condoms to people who are in such a situation is good advice. But with the virus spreading slowly, the average chance that one's next sexual contact would be with a highly infectious person is very small. Under these circumstances, to make a substantial difference to the overall prevalence of infection would require virtually the entire population using condoms for almost every instance of intercourse.

about the "ethics" of monitoring the blood supply and preventing contamination of transfused blood or blood products with the AIDS virus—but really they were about the finances involved.* And there were controversies over the "messages" that might be sent to users of illegal drugs if access to clean needles and syringes were allowed. The discussion was about risk and reproved behavior.

Other than the French scandal over blood banking, the matter of blood was less discussed outside the United States. Still, in Britain, the Netherlands, France, Germany, Switzerland, Australia, and Canada, at least at times, it was more acceptable to talk about practical interventions to prevent users of illicit drugs from harming themselves by injecting HIV-contaminated blood. These included the deliberate distribution of sterile needles and syringes and the provision of heroin-substitution drugs that did not need to be injected, primarily methadone. Later, safe-injecting rooms opened where users could obtain sterile equipment and inject in clean surroundings with medical attention on hand in case of overdose. Harm minimization, or harm reduction, as the latter interventions came to be called collectively, gradually gained in popularity. But in America, to view drug use as normal, if ill-advised, would have been to see blood-borne AIDS spread as a public-health nuisance that could be dealt with pragmatically and without rhetoric, along the lines of measles prevention by vaccine. It would have eliminated the questions of imprudence and excess, and thereby would have conflicted with profoundly American fears that helped write the story of the new epidemic. Talking about AIDS in terms other than an excess of appetite or a failure of impulse control would have silenced the voices of those who clamored for

---

*When circuit court judge Richard Posner ruled against the plaintiffs in a class-action lawsuit filed against the National Hemophilia Foundation, a consumer group, and four companies that fractionate blood into transfusable products for hemophiliacs, on the grounds that they failed to protect recipients of blood products from infection with HIV, he wrote that the suit could throw the blood-banking industry into bankruptcy.

civil rights for gay Americans in part on the grounds that homosexuals are a minority targeted by a behavioral disease. And it would have undercut the moralists for whom AIDS was not merely a disease but a meaningful tragedy that proved that sexual contact between men is a violation of nature.

—ɯ—

The culture cooperated with the coding of AIDS as a failure of prudence. Popular art and media rhetoric amplified the point. By the late 1980s it had become clear that AIDS could be depicted in the popular media of film or television only if it occurred in an "innocent" transfusion recipient or a child infected in utero (Britain's Princess Anne had made the distinction explicit at a world meeting of health ministers held in London in 1988, publicly lamenting the "tragedy" of AIDS's "innocent victims": transfusion recipients and children infected in the womb). The other sufferers, the tremendous majority who acquired AIDS through lust for satisfaction or euphoria (or just relief), were never seen, a reminder that those who are not innocent are (as Susan Sontag reminded us) guilty. Not until 1990 do homosexual AIDS sufferers appear on-screen as sympathetic characters, in Norman René's film *Longtime Companion*, and they are portrayed as wealthy and handsome. In Jonathan Demme's *Philadelphia* (1993), which aimed to be a "mainstream" (code for "not gay") film, the homosexual character afflicted with AIDS is again well-to-do (a lawyer) and good-looking (he was played by Tom Hanks). In such elusive examples, there wasn't room for the equivalent of the instructive horror and general promise of, say, the Isenheim altarpiece, or for confrontation with our own prejudices.

In visual works meant for a wide audience, AIDS was not just sanitized but recoded: it was a misfortune suffered by the innocent at the hands of the beautiful. In a reprise of the early-twentieth-century sexual-hygiene campaigns connecting syphilis to the vampirism of

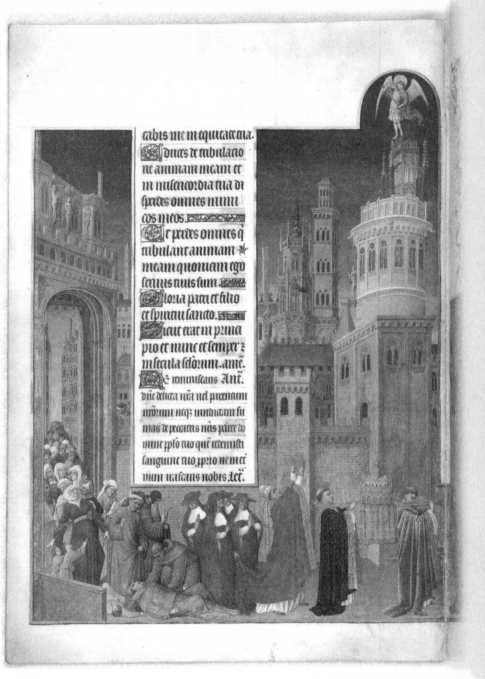

Figure 1. *The Procession of Pope Gregory the Great (St. Gregory) for the Cessation of the Plague in Rome.* Limbourg Brothers (fifteenth century). The illuminated miniature, the left half of a larger piece, is from the *Très Riches Heures du Duc de Berry: The Penitential Psalms* (Ms. 65, f. 71 verso), 1416. Musée Condé, Chantilly, France.

Photo: R.G. Ojeda. Réunion des Musées Nationaux/Art Resource, NY.

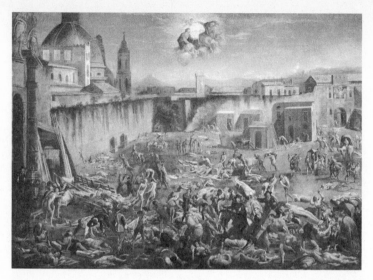

Figure 2. *The Piazza del Mercatello in Naples During the Plague of 1656*, painted by Micco Spadaro (Domenico Gargiulo). The scene shows the devastation wrought by the plague outbreak, with officials directing the cleanup of corpses. Museo di San Martino, Naples, Italy. *Scala/Ministerio per I Beni e le Attività Culturali/Art Resource, NY.*

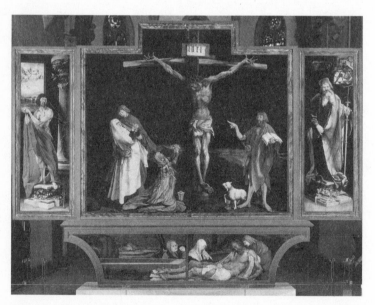

Figure 3. *The Isenheim Altarpiece.* Mathias Grünewald (1455–1528). France. Grünewald's altarpiece, executed for the abbots of the Order of St. Anthony in Isenheim in 1505 and completed between 1512 and 1516, was an emblem of the possibility of salvation through faith. St. Anthony in the desert appears in the rightmost panel, the centerpiece shows the crucifixion, and St. Sebastian is depicted at left. Musée d'Unterlinden, Colmar. *Scala/Art Resource, NY.*

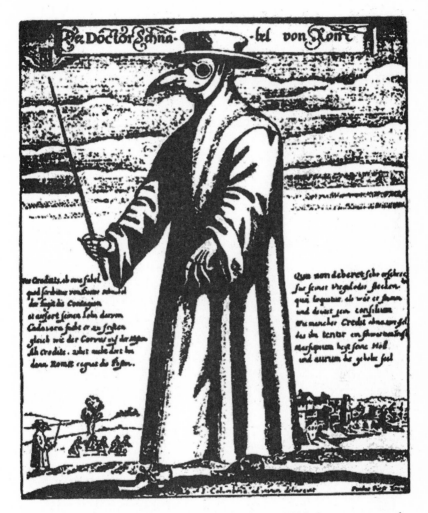

Figure 4. *Doktor Schnabel of Rome*, Paulus Fürst, 1656. An engraving of a plague doctor in customary dress. The birdlike mask was meant to help filter plague-infested air.

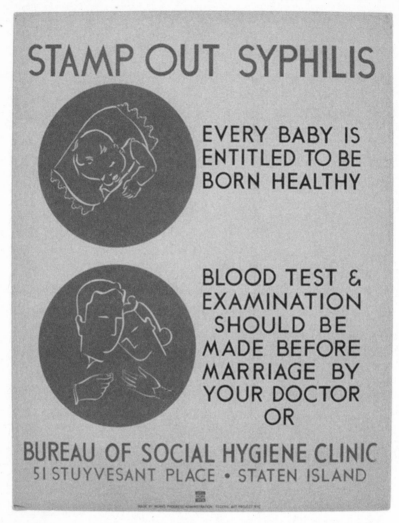

Figure 5. *Stamp Out Syphilis*. Posters like this one were produced by the Bureau of Social Hygiene, part of the Progressive movement's effort to eliminate venereal disease and improve public morals. The Bureau of Social Hygiene, established in New York City in 1913, was dedicated to "the study, amelioration, and prevention of those social conditions, crimes, and diseases which adversely affect the well-being of society, with special reference to prostitution and the evils associated therewith."

The National Library of Medicine, History of Medicine Division, Prints and Photographs Collection, http://wwwihm.nlm.nih.gov/.

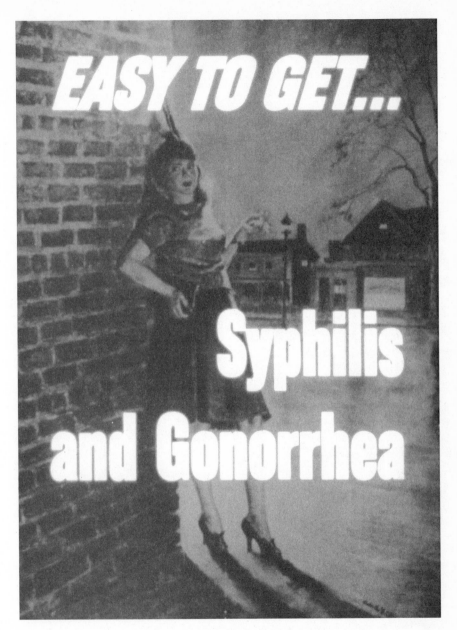

Figure 6. *Easy to Get: Syphilis and Gonorrhea.* Charles Casa, 1940. The title on the image obviously refers to both the availability of the woman and the diseases she supposedly carries. This poster is typical of ones produced for mid-twentieth-century anti-VD campaigns in the United States.

The National Library of Medicine, History of Medicine Division, Prints and Photographs Collection, http://wwwihm.nlm.nih.gov/.

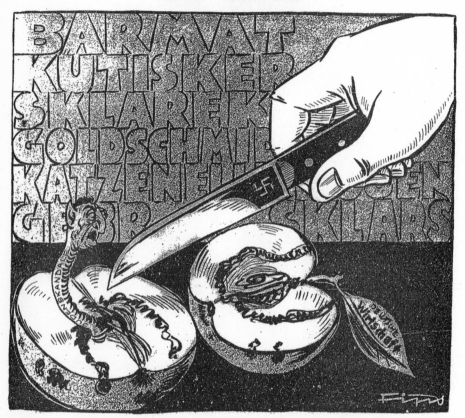

Figure 7. *Der Wurm.* In this cartoon from the Nazi propaganda publication *Der Stürmer*, Jews are the cause of the decay of the fruitful German economy. The caption reads, "The Worm: Where something is rotten, the Jew is the cause."

German Propaganda Archive site, http://www.calvin.edu/academic/cas/gpa/sturm28.htm, courtesy of Randall Bytwerk.

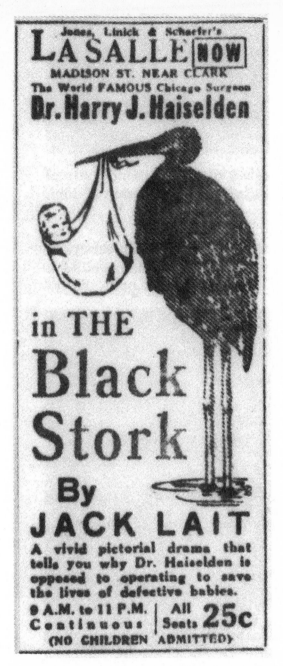

Figure 8. *The Black Stork.* This graphic advertising the film *The Black Stork,* whose plot promoted eugenic themes, appeared in the April 2, 1917, *Chicago Tribune.*

© 1917 Chicago Tribune. All rights reserved. Used by permission and protected by the copyright laws of the United States. The printing, copying redistribution, or retransmission of the material without express written permission is prohibited.

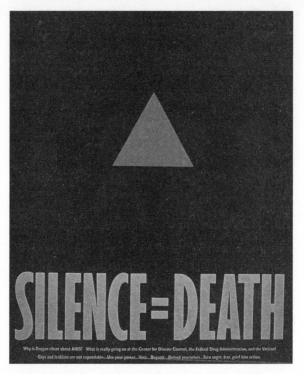

Figure 9. Silence = Death Project, 1986. This image, produced by the Silence = Death Project, was later sent to the activist alliance ACT-UP and became an icon of the AIDS world.

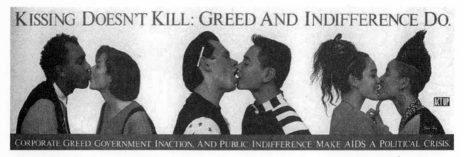

Figure 10. *Kissing Doesn't Kill*, 1989. Designed by the activist art collective Gran Fury, *Kissing Doesn't Kill* highlighted the effects of homophobia and criticized U.S. government's sluggish response to AIDS. The image appeared on a postcard whose obverse read "Corporate Greed, Government Inaction, and Public Indifference Make AIDS a Political Crisis."

the debonair, looks do kill in films about AIDS. In the 1993 made-for-television film version of *And the Band Played On* (directed by Roger Spottiswoode), the Canadian airline steward Gaetan Dugas, popularized in the book version as the man who brought the AIDS virus to the United States, appears as a modern-day Dracula: handsome and well dressed, smoking a cigarette (the devil's sign, at least in the States), and speaking heavily accented English (thus: foreign). And, true to both the film's narrative and the new thinking, Dugas refuses to be cautious. The matter of safety becomes paramount.

Two images forbidden in popular media, sexual love between men and the disfigurement of AIDS, were brought forward for sympathetic audiences in other forms of art. The visual art of plagues past had shown the epidemic as abnormal, the suffering as stylized (and meant to induce guilt and thereby amplify the viewer's piety), the causes as external and essentially inscrutable. Plague art had been the art of the innocent, beseeching God for favor, in response to an epidemic that was everybody's business. AIDS art responded to an epidemic that was deemed by many to be the problem of a few. It was the art of the culpable. In an epidemic in which cause was synonymous with riskiness, gay men were implicitly guilty—of harboring impulses that could lead to social destruction.

In photography, graphic art, and other forms of visual expression, gay artists countered the implication of guilt. They sought to depict same-sex love as essentially beautiful, eliminating the distinctions between homosexual and heterosexual love, and stripping the suffering of AIDS victims of its stylizations. In keeping with the national decision about the problem of AIDS, they aimed additionally to recode the cause of the epidemic not as imprudence or violation of norms but as a lack of information. In 1987, the Silence = Death Project wrapped art, education, and gay liberation into a single image that would become iconic: the pink triangle, alluding to Nazi concentration camps, above the phrase "Silence = Death." It made graphic the allegation that government indifference made AIDS tantamount to a Holocaust visited on gays. The artful elision of text in favor of the "=" sign, placed under an equilateral triangle, neatly suggested a mathematical notation—perhaps meant to allude further to the famous technological refinement of the machinery of Nazi killing (see figure 9).

The art collective Gran Fury produced the "Kissing Doesn't Kill" image in 1989, playing against fears of racial and sexual miscegenation and implicitly linking ignorance of AIDS education with capitalist excess (see figure 10). Constructed as a postcard whose obverse read "Corporate Greed, Government Inaction, and Public Indifference Make AIDS a Political Crisis," the image showed three kissing couples: one male-female, one male-male, and one female-female and comprising varying mixes of ethnic background. It was later made into a poster that appeared on buses in New York City. As with "Silence = Death," this work demands more of the viewer than art conventionally does: more than merely discomfiting, it explicitly enjoins the viewer to act. Further, it suggests that owning up to one's sexuality is itself an act of defiance.

—m—

The behavioral turn might have eliminated race from the epidemic story—after all, when looking for the source of an epidemic inside ourselves, within our impulses and our decisions to act on them or not, it would seem that externals like skin color might not matter. Yet race pervaded the new epidemic from early on. AIDS served to bring out imagined distinctions between blacks and whites. Imputing a behavioral basis to AIDS and then seeing it as a racial disease, Americans made AIDS available for the effort to assign a biological foundation to race.

With a higher prevalence of AIDS in some black populations, it was easy for certain people to suppose that a characteristic set of behaviors that black Americans engage in made them especially vulnerable to infection with the virus. By 1988, the Department of Health and Human Services was looking into specialized AIDS education campaigns for black (and also Hispanic) Americans—the assumption being that minority groups would not be served by advice produced for "mainstream" Americans. Thus, national policy on AIDS implicitly recognized the racial presumption that there is something distinctly wrong with the behavior of people considered to be nonwhite.

Gayness, already divided from the "mainstream," was itself subdivided by race. The racial division took place with the consent of gay activists. Initial funding for new education campaigns that were supposedly specific for African American homosexual men went to a gay organization, the National Task Force for AIDS Prevention. The behavioral turn linked with prejudices about race to fragment the nascent organization of gay men (and women). Separate racial camps formed, competing for attention and funding.

Further cementing the link between race and behavior, there were apocryphal allegations about the "down-low." Articles in the early 2000s claimed that black homosexual men had no identification with gayness and tended to live closeted lives, often as married men who engaged in sexual liaisons with other men. The DL phenomenon, as it came to be called, supposedly created a special risk for both black gay men and the women who were their partners. The myth of specialness was promoted by the CDC, which posted reports on its Web site about the down-low. The CDC reports carefully rejected the notion that the DL had anything to do with race, but they went on to mention connections between the DL and the "African American community" that could only validate suspicions of racial separateness around sexuality and play on Western fears of black Africa in general and African AIDS in particular. The CDC asserted that "there are no data to confirm or refute publicized accounts of HIV risk behavior associated with these [i.e., DL] men" but nonetheless listed detailed "sexual risk factors associated with being on the down-low."

Men in Western cultures have long taken male lovers but stayed married. In the early seventeenth century, prosecutions for sodomy declined and, at least for the upper classes, liaisons between men were open secrets. By the 1830s, even in middle-class America, there were homosexual cruising grounds in New York City and all-male clubs understood to be venues for sex. Homosexuality remained a practice that, although stigmatized (and technically illegal), both single and married men engaged in during the twentieth century. The claim, in a twenty-first-century news story, that the down-low was new and uniquely dangerous for black Americans was an opportunistic attempt by journalists to create news where there was none. And it had a more pernicious and implicitly racial effect: it suggested that there was something about blackness that resisted gay liberation. You can be gay and "out" if you are white, it signaled, but blacks are unable or unwilling to claim the newly recognized right to a sexual identity.

The use of AIDS to biologize race extended neatly into the American War on Drugs. Always fundamentally a war against drug users more than against drug use, the national campaign coupled with AIDS anxiety to anathematize black men. Given the common, albeit incorrect, belief that drug addicts were generally black, AIDS risk was widely understood to imply that black Americans bore some special responsibility for the disease. Race was like gayness in this respect, since homosexuals were also held responsible. But, especially after black gays had been marginalized by the assertion that they needed special prevention programs, gayness and blackness were distinct variables of "risk."

As with syphilis, AIDS played into fears of the sexual black man. Anxieties elicited by black male sexual license served to highlight other stereotypes as well. A white girl who had had condomless intercourse with a black man infected with the AIDS virus was a victim, and her victimhood was understood to be the consequence of "poor choices" or "low self-esteem," even if she was also understood to have been stupid or injudicious (and whether or not she actually contracted AIDS through this act). The black man who had sex with her was deemed capable of sexual "depravity."

In cases where many white women had had sex with an HIV-infected black man, the man would be fashioned by the media as a "monster," a "lethal lothario," a "walking epidemic," or "the bogey-man incarnate." The 1997 case of Nushawn Williams, a young black man from Brooklyn who violated the decorum of race and place by moving to Jamestown in upstate New York and having sex with dozens of girls and women there, became grounds for a media festival. It turned out that Williams carried the AIDS virus and that thirteen of the women who named him as a sex partner were infected, as was a child (not Williams's) born to one of the women. Because the women named a total of eighty-five sexual contacts they'd had, some of whom were drug users, it was never certain how many women actually had been infected by Williams. Of some 1,400 people who came forward for HIV testing in Chautauqua County after the case was publicized, only one was positive. There had been no "one-man epidemic," as some media stories claimed. Yet Williams's name was released to the public by the state's Department of Health, the only instance in which the state's HIV Confidentiality Law was ever violated.

The media crafted the monster story into a morality tale of willful perfidy on the part of a demonic criminal and of naïveté on the part of the community from which his so-called victims were drawn. Williams was prosecuted (he pleaded guilty and served eight years in penitentiary for reckless endangerment and statutory rape), although it was never certain that Williams had understood that he carried a virulent germ, might infect others, and should always use a condom in order to make sure he did not transmit a dangerous infection. Echoing the Williams case, in 2004 a black man in Olympia, Washington, was convicted of first-degree assault for knowingly exposing seventeen white women to the AIDS virus (five became infected). A judge sentenced him to 178 years in prison. A Canadian court in 2005 allowed first-degree murder charges to be brought against a black immigrant with

HIV who had had sexual intercourse with white women, two of whom contracted AIDS and died. The man was convicted and sentenced to fifty-six months in prison in 2007.

AIDS does not make every black man who has sex with multiple white women a monster, though. Fears of miscegenation can have nuances. After basketball star Magic Johnson went public with the news that he had the AIDS virus in November 1991, sports fans and journalists were lavish with praise. "Anyone is vulnerable to deep tragedy," one sportswriter observed, before pointing out that Johnson was a "fine and courageous man." Another, reporting Johnson's "explanation" that before he had married he had "accommodated" as many women as he could, called Johnson "a victim, not a hero." There was widespread sympathy for Johnson's "plight." Johnson dispelled rumors of homosexual liaisons by averring, again and again, that he was certain that he contracted the AIDS virus through sex with a woman. He claimed to be searching for the woman responsible for infecting him, but, he told the *Financial Post*, "most people are coming up negative."

That the "people" in question in Johnson's case were women was not pursued. Nor was the question of who infected whom. Whereas Nushawn Williams's women had been victims, and a few were extensively profiled in articles published about the incident, Magic Johnson's women were faceless and nameless—just scenery on the stage on which the sports star acted. Many stories repeated the claim by Wilt Chamberlain, a basketball star from an earlier era, that he had had sex with 20,000 women—implying that Johnson, who made no claims about numbers of sexual liaisons, had been either more modest in his sexual ambitions or merely less boastful, but in any case reminding us that physical prowess and personal magnetism need not be restricted to the basketball court. The pious praise of Johnson drowned out the similarities between his story and that of Williams or the other, nonsuperstar black men who were prosecuted.

While the difference between the Williams case and the Johnson case might have more to do with privilege than race, the public shaming and then equally public exoneration of the "victimized" women involved in the former was so distant from the utter invisibility of the women involved in the latter that we are left to conclude that the AIDS story is malleable in the hands of whomever happens to be telling it. When the epidemic, rewritten as a calamity of male misbehavior and carrying overtones of race, bumped up against fame, the women who collaborated in a star male athlete's alleged sexual misbehavior disappeared.

THE PERSISTENT THEME OF BEHAVIOR

The us-versus-them rhetoric of AIDS—the attempt to vilify homosexuals or indict homosexuality itself—was evident from the outset. But the new thinking was more complex than that. With AIDS, epidemic thinking eventually came to embrace us-versus-us even more than us-versus-them. The internal struggles of the culture, the tragic Apollonian-Dionysian dance by which we deliberate over what is the right thing to do (sexual abstemiousness versus sex education, for instance) while questioning whether our appetites have been fully sated, led us to replace the clear divisions offered by national origin with identities based on affinity. The ambivalence over appetite moved us to substitute "community," as in "the gay community" or "the African American community," for neighborhood or commons—as if there could be only one such community, as if anyone would know where to find it, and as if anyone who met the requisite qualification would be embraced there. The us-versus-us underlay of the contemporary epidemic allowed people to distance themselves from their fellows. In the name of AIDS, society separated the lascivious and the voracious from the so-called mainstream.

The paranoid mentality that came to define our reaction to AIDS was plainly evident in February 2005, when the health commissioner of New York City raised a public alarm about a single new case of AIDS.

New York had been accustomed to AIDS illness and death. By 1983, the city was already producing half the AIDS cases in the nation; more than a thousand New Yorkers were diagnosed with AIDS that year. Through 1983 and '84, the rate at which new cases appeared was doubling every fifteen to twenty months. Proportionately, more San Franciscans would die of AIDS than in any other U.S. city, but New York was unequaled for the sheer number of AIDS deaths. About one out of every seven American deaths from AIDS was recorded in New York City. By 2005, a quarter-century after the first cases were noted, the AIDS virus had been responsible for the deaths of 84,000 New Yorkers.

That February, summoning the media for a televised press conference, the health commissioner informed the public that a "city resident [has been] diagnosed with [a] rare strain of multi-drug resistant HIV that rapidly progresses to AIDS." The commissioner explained that the case was a man in his mid-forties who "reported multiple male sex partners and unprotected anal intercourse," and said that the man often used a popular drug reputed to be associated with sexual recklessness. The occurrence, the commissioner declared, should be a "wake-up call to . . . men who have sex with men." Gay spokesmen chimed in, urging sexual "responsibility" on their compeers.

A few days after the alert, the health commissioner, conceding that he wasn't sure "whether this [occurrence] is of tremendous scientific importance," asserted that the alert was needed because "people have not dealt with HIV as if it were an epidemic [and we] are trying to change that." The main focus of the alert was an advisory to "the community of men who have sex with men," he adumbrated. Such men "successfully reduced [their] risk of HIV in the 1980s" and had to "do so again to stop the devastation of HIV/AIDS and the spread of drug-resistant strains." That is, the onus would be on the community to bring the behavior of its members into line with the standard. It was an injunction with the overtones of a sermon. Mayor Michael Bloomberg reached more explicitly into church language, telling the *New York Times* that unprotected sex was "just a sin in our society."

The media attention that followed the press conference, the public concern, and the sense that both the case and the announcement were extraordinary were, taken together, an emblem of how the epidemic had become a social event defined by the way we talk about the event itself. It demonstrated the appeal of the notion that each community is responsible for curbing the appetites of its members in order to protect the public.

The curbing of appetites seemed more important than the facts. The AIDS case that triggered the commissioner's panic was not, as he had claimed, the first person with AIDS to have both a rapidly progressing and multiply drug-resistant infection: four years earlier, two such cases had been reported in Vancouver. Both of the earlier cases had responded to treatment, as the New York case later did. Similarly, in 2008, when the Swiss National Commission on AIDS said that HIV-infected people who had undergone treatment, showed very low levels of circulating virus, and had no other genital infections might judiciously have sex without condoms, professionals in the AIDS field decried the announcement. AIDS offers a rationale by which we can always enjoin others to be abstemious.

THE WORLD'S EPIDEMIC

AIDS is the epidemic of our time, partly because it allows us to express feelings that would otherwise be unspeakable. Misgivings about sexual excess or sexual difference can be expressed in the sanitized form of decrying risky behavior and may seem to be not a moral stand but a health claim. Discomfort with the human appetite for euphoria or ecstasy can be stated as an appeal to suppress illicit drug use or sexual promiscuity and may seem like a principled policy position rather than fear of the irrational. Dismay at the way economic policies have preserved a wide disparity in wealth between the world's rich and poor can be recoded as concern about the adequacy of aid to the unfortunate victims of the epidemic in Africa or Asia. And AIDS has made risk central to our view of ourselves, giving voice to a deep anxiety about whether the modern world, which seems to have broken with the past, harbors unprecedented dangers.

AIDS affects many millions, yet its prevalence cannot explain why it dominates the discussion of global health. According to the United Nations Joint Programme on HIV/AIDS (UNAIDS), more than 33 million people were living with the causative virus at the end of 2007, and more than 2 million die of AIDS each year (cumulatively, between 67 million and 80 million Africans will have died of AIDS by 2025). Malaria (500 million cases each year, more than 1 million annual deaths) and tuberculosis (8.8 million new cases each year, 1.6 million deaths) register far less powerfully. AIDS is the epidemic of our time because it provides the lens through which we see our era and the language we use to talk about our world.

In 1989, the late Susan Sontag wondered, hopefully, whether a day would come when even AIDS, then still "the disease most fraught with meaning," would "become just an illness." AIDS ought to be a commonplace illness now, not much different from malaria, TB, or the other diseases (measles, diarrhea, sleeping sickness, dengue, and others) that ravage the poor countries of the world and affect us in the rich ones, albeit far less so. Yet AIDS remains exceptional. When Peter Piot, director of UNAIDS, in a speech to the 2006 World AIDS Conference, exhorted the throng to "maintain the exceptionality of AIDS on political agendas," he meant that to let AIDS be anything other than extraordinary might interfere with the world's view of UNAIDS as a heroic army. When organizations say they are "fighting" AIDS, they mean they see themselves as modern-day versions of Docteur Rieux from Camus's The Plague, selflessly helping to alleviate the human costs of disaster. If AIDS were not exceptional, the world might fail to see today's AIDS "warriors" as heroic, might miss the distinction between them and, for instance, those Public Health Service physicians who failed to help the help-less in Tuskegee. "The end of AIDS exceptionality would spell the end of protected funding for antiretroviral therapy, of commitment to harm reduction for injecting drug use, of sex education in schools, of billions for the AIDS response," said Piot. "The real threat is too little recognition—not too much!—that AIDS is an exceptional cri-sis and worsening threat."

Given that the overwhelming bulk of AIDS cases occur in very poor countries, to claim that AIDS is, and must remain, extraordi-nary is to throw up hands in resignation and accept as normal—not exceptional—an economic status quo of gross inequity. The contin-uance of AIDS as a disaster of plaguelike proportions would be im-possible except for the gap between the enormous capacity of wealthy countries to protect the health of their citizens and the des-titution of poor countries. To allow AIDS to seem extraordinary, un-precedented, and unfathomable is to pretend that before AIDS it had not been true that half the population would die before the age of forty in parts of Africa while in Western Europe and Japan half the population will live past eighty. It is to say that there is not much to be done about a status quo in which possibility is a com-modity whose availability is sharply divided. Perhaps the urge to keep AIDS exceptional comes in part from the desire to use AIDS as a lever by which some of the wealth of Europe and the United States could be pried loose to help the poorer nations of the world. But keeping AIDS extraordinary also allows the powerful to con-tinue to claim that the division between haves and have-nots (or, equally, between live-longs and die-youngs) is unusual, that it is not a result of the very ordinary failure of the affluent to act justly in the face of a long-standing disparity in wealth and power. AIDS is so in-herently aberrant, we are meant to understand, that we need only "fight" AIDS. We need not attend to the realities that make AIDS catastrophic in some parts of the world and just another treatable disease at home. The appeal made by the director of UNAIDS for maintaining the exceptionality of AIDS testifies to the investment of even our era's most prominent international agencies, and even people who advocate human rights, in prolonging the inequity that keeps some people's lives short and their choices limited. It grants opportunities to businesses that sell products to help people to "reduce their risk." It ensures that AIDS agencies stay in business. And it keeps the focus on everyone's behavior—the germ within.

Chapter 7

MANAGING THE IMAGINED EPIDEMIC

Our concern with history . . . is a concern with
preformed images already imprinted on our
brains, images at which we keep staring while
the truth lies elsewhere, away from it all, somewhere as yet undiscovered.

—W. G. Sebald, Austerlitz

By the mid-1990s exhortations to transfer our fears onto disease
epidemics that had not yet happened abounded. By 1994,
"emerging infections" had become a buzz phrase in disease policy.
Two important books published that year were instrumental in
arousing concern. In *The Hot Zone*, Richard Preston recounted a
real incident in which the Ebola virus was transmitted among animals in a lab in the Washington, D.C., area and spread within the
community. Response to the book resonated with fears of dangers
emerging from within—from within the lab, but also from within
our modern living arrangements, which allow labs that conduct experiments on pathogenic germs to be located near populous suburbs.

Ebola, a virus associated with outbreaks of severe hemorrhagic
fever in Sudan and Zaire (now Democratic Republic of the Congo)
in the 1970s, seemed particularly fearsome. Fatality rates in Ebola

outbreaks have been astronomical—higher than those of nineteenth-century cholera outbreaks and reaching near 90 percent. To this day, Ebola remains a frightening mystery. Unlike the panic-inducing infections of the past, Ebola seems to have few if any human carriers. It isn't clear how or why outbreaks happen or where the virus resides between outbreaks. Presumably, it infects forest animals, but exactly which remains unknown. No human deaths occurred in the incident described in *The Hot Zone*; the strain of Ebola in question was not one that infects humans. But the event reminded us that viruses are far from conquered.

Laurie Garrett's *The Coming Plague* made the connection between so-called emerging infections and human error immediate. Garrett's book warned of "newly emerging diseases in a world out of balance." Carefully documenting the appearance of previously unheard-of conditions (toxic shock syndrome, Legionnaires' disease, AIDS, and Ebola among them), the book sounded an alarm about the modern-day failure to acknowledge the complexity and danger of nature itself.

While the two books were stirring attention, the CDC was sounding its own alarm. In *Addressing Emerging Infectious Disease Threats: A Prevention Strategy for the United States*, published in April 1994, the CDC drew directly on the fear of AIDS and the notion, prevalent by then, that danger lurks inside the very systems we have developed to protect ourselves. The CDC report played the common AIDS-era theme of the dangers of indifference to threats from within.

As a consequence of changes in society, technology, and the environment, pathogens evolve or spread, and the spectrum of infectious diseases expands. Emerging infections, such as human immunodeficiency virus (HIV)/acquired immunodeficiency syndrome (AIDS), illustrate that no nation can be complacent regarding human vulnerability to microorganisms in the environment.

In the view expressed in the report, the difficulty in preventing emerging infections could be linked to the tale of the new epidemic—

one that was traceable to imprudence and especially to the dangers of sex and sexuality, female sexuality most of all. When the report noted that enrollment in day-care facilities had increased "as more mothers of young children have entered the work force," it offered a subtle form of the customary accusation that women are failing in their duty to marry and stay home and harked back to reports from the 1920s about girls catching (and spreading) TB because they left home to work in factories or offices and preferred short skirts to long dresses.

The report did make valid points about disease control: it emphasized that disease threats arise in part because of "economic impoverishment, war or civil conflict, population growth and migration, [and] urban decay." But the list of contributing factors was filled with the anxieties of modern life. Emerging infections, it argued, come about not only because of changes in organisms or the environment (the report acknowledged global warming and deforestation) but also because of organ and tissue transplantation, new medical devices, globalization of food supplies, outdoor recreation, sexual behavior, illicit drug use, diet, and food preparation. In other words, modern living helps the pathogens that lurk deep in our society to emerge and harm us. In 1995, with the supposed threat of emergence in the news, the CDC sought to keep it on the front lines of science by establishing a new journal for research articles called *Emerging Infectious Diseases.*

A government agency like CDC has a certain interest in asserting that the public is complacent. In the mid-'90s, just as AIDS was coming under control and the CDC's work was receding from the headlines, the emerging-infections initiative channeled new financing to federal health agencies. Total emerging-infections funding to the National Institute for Allergy and Infectious Diseases (just one of the National Institutes of Health) increased thirtyfold, from $47 million in 1994 to more than $1.7 billion in 2005. The CDC budget for emerging infections (independent of monies for control of known infectious problems) had climbed to more than $125 million by 2008; that the proposed 2009 federal budget will cut that amount by one-fifth has elicited consternation among infectious-disease scientists.

As the scare over bioterrorism of the early 2000s would demonstrate, warnings about health crises have political uses. Anxiety about human appetites and fixed memories of long-ago plagues set the stage, as did a presumption, articulated in books and editorials at the turn of the twenty-first century, that the human capacity for mayhem had so greatly expanded that official agencies could no longer prevent the gravest of man-made catastrophes. The lack of confidence in government capacities to defend us was, by then, supported by a belief that U.S. officials might have successfully prevented the 9/11 attacks if they had had sufficient warning—a supposition not consistent with the facts, as the September 11 Commission revealed. But, as with TSS and Legionnaires' disease, the facts were more easily dismissed than the force of the narrative. By late 2001, feeling vulnerable, the public reacted hysterically. Officials eager to restore their legitimacy as defenders of the public's health and safety rode the wave.

THE BIOTERRORISM SCARE

In 2002 President George Bush's multimillion-dollar Project BioShield program was announced. The funding for the abortive smallpox-vaccination endeavor was part of BioShield, but the program didn't end when the vaccination initiative went belly up. BioShield allocated more than $10 billion for bioterrorism prevention and biosecurity by mid-2004. "Biopreparedness" became a watchword as the public-health apparatus was recruited to promote and maintain fear. As the terms of America's foreign policy switched from war on terrorism to war on terror, the agencies formerly charged with controlling disease became agents of the maintenance of fear. The Department of Health and Human Services, which houses the CDC and the National Institutes of Health, was allocated $1.5 billion in 2003–2004 alone to promote "biodefense medical research and development." The BioShield program supported a state of dread by preparing, prominently and publicly, for a disaster that was highly improbable yet, it implied, inevitable.

An aspect of the biosecurity program that seemed bent on keeping fear foremost in the public's mind was the staging of U.S.-led international "biopreparedness exercises." One organizer of the Atlantic Storm exercise, which took place in January 2005, asserted that "this is not science fiction. The age of bioterror is now." The claim that bioterrorism was happening, or might happen, was at odds with the facts, but again the narrative moved forward with its *own* facts. In the Atlantic Storm scenario, an Islamic terrorist group grew smallpox virus in a lab that the terrorists had disguised as a brewery in Klagenfurt, Austria, before releasing the virus on the subways in Rotterdam and Warsaw, in the airports in Frankfurt and Los Angeles, in New York City's Penn Station, and at the Grand Bazaar in Istanbul. The plot was made up, but the planning that went into it was real and considerable, and the language the biosecurity planners used to describe the exercise was designed to stir up terrors of nightmarish illness and civil unrest.

It's not that the bioterrorism scenarios are implausible. Anything can happen. Rarely, that has included biological warfare—although its record of producing epidemic disease is thin. The infamous Unit 731 of the Japanese Imperial Army created some severe outbreaks of plague and cholera in its efforts to subjugate the occupied Chinese population during the Second World War. In 1984, more than 750 people in Oregon contracted diarrhea by eating from salad bars that had been contaminated with the bacterium *Salmonella typhimurium* by disgruntled members of a religious cult. The five deaths in the anthrax event of 2001 represent the only mortality in purposely created outbreaks outside wartime.

The truth is, the very plausibility of scenarios involving contaminated reservoirs, viruses sprayed in a ventilating system, aerosolized bacteria released in a subway car at rush hour, and the like renders them innocuous. The great calamities are always, and have always been, unforeseeable and unimaginable until the moment they begin. The terror inspired by the Black Death, the religious furor of the cholera outbreaks, and the pained resignation to fate at the time of the Spanish Flu were not elicited by the suddenness of the epidemic's onset and the excessive mortality alone: they were also expressions of existential dread. To witness the material of dark fantasies and nightmares in real life is to realize that nature is capable of unpredictable, incoherent violence.

The core fallacy of bioterrorism preparedness is that, when it comes to the unforeseeable event, humans have never outdone nature. The Spanish Flu of 1918 killed at least twice as many people as did the First World War. Ten times more people were killed by smallpox in the course of the twentieth century than died in the Second World War—even including the Holocaust and all other civilian deaths in the wartime total. It does not minimize the horrors that men and machines have wreaked on humankind to acknowledge that our man-made slaughters never reach the awfulness of nature's. It is a waste of time and energy to prepare for what we can't foresee, and it is a lie to pretend, as the biopreparedness promoters have, that we can see what we cannot. The biopreparedness hysteria blinds us to the imperative of civic life. Since anything can happen, it makes sense to prepare for the *probable* perils (blizzards in winter, drought in summer, the annual outbreak of flu) and plan for the *present* danger (malaria in equatorial regions, antibiotic-resistant bacteria in urban hospitals, and so forth)—because there's nothing to be gained by trying to prepare for the unlikely and unforeseeable.

HEALTH OFFICIALS AS SOOTHSAYERS

As the bioterrorism scare illustrates, we use epidemics to invest health officials with a dual authority: to inform us about dangers that are not apparent to the unschooled eye (strangers bearing weaponized germs, for instance) and to direct our defenses against these threats. In the past, authorities made recommendations for prevention; their job was to defend against the real threat (the suspected dangers were the clergy's purview). AIDS altered the role of the health official. With AIDS, the epidemic was inapparent in essence—it was understood to be a matter of viral spread and latent infectivity. When AIDS became an epidemic of riskiness, of untoward behavior and dangerous acts waiting to happen, we began to expect our health officials to identify what was risky. We empowered them to educate the public about risk behavior and advise us as to what to do, what not to do, and whom to avoid. The invisible epidemic, the outbreak of risk or the possibility of risk, is necessarily an imagined one. We appoint officials to do the imagining for us.

Asking our health officials to divine what will harm the public and to recommend evasive action puts them in a curious role. They must act like wizards. When health officials were supposed to defend against obvious outbreaks, they had to take explicit action to control the spread of contagion. Their programs were sometimes morally suspect (the U.S. Marine Hospital Service official Joseph Kinyoun's demand that Chinese people be quarantined during the San Francisco plague outbreak of 1900 comes to mind), but they were responding to real dangers. To do nothing in the face of an evidently fierce outbreak constituted obvious misfeasance on the part of a public official. But now that an epidemic allegedly is hidden and its cause supposedly impossible to identify (but somehow camouflaged within our social arrangements or our behavior), officials are not supposed to respond. That would be to act too late. Instead, they are supposed to foresee, as though with crystal ball in hand.

When health officials play the role of soothsayers, they are granted a path to legitimating their power—a way to make it seem as if they are doing something valuable even while they do nothing. If enough people are frightened by bioterrorism, then it will be an act of civic virtue when a health official reminds us to duct-tape our windows against aerosolized germs. The official will have answered our need to lessen anxiety. But she will not have done anything to make us safer.

It is naturally impossible to fix a problem that has not yet occurred. Health agencies cannot curtail an epidemic of smallpox created purposely by "bioterrorists" because it does not exist. But they can claim to have identified such nonevents as real threats and then, once they have prescribed preventive action, every day that the improbable epidemic does not happen serves to legitimate their diagnosis and prescriptions. Public-health policy becomes a magic show, the official engaging in legerdemain and the public—the conjurer's audience—agreeing to believe that the official has succeeded in pulling off an inexplicable trick. When we watch Atlantic Storm with its pretend attacks on the subways, or any other bioterrorism drill, and then see no man-made epidemic take place afterward, it is easy to conclude that the nonevent was a result of the officials' vigilance, their "biopreparedness." And in a climate of hyped-up fears of new, hidden dangers, who would dare to say that the preparations were useless?

THE OBESITY SCARE

When officials invoke the specter of bioterrorists poisoning the water supply, they play on ancient fears of foreigners and modern anxieties about civic disruption. Biopreparedness translates our anxieties about modern life into fears of the improbable and undetectable threat. But what if the threat is allegedly within us—not just within the mechanics of modernity, as with TSS or Legionnaires', or with the observable risk behavior we have been taught to revile, like needle sharing, but inside our own bodies? Most recently, the risk that abides inside us has become the focus of our dread. As with biopreparedness, the so-called epidemic of obesity plays on fantasies of mayhem and misgivings about our own habits. When the public is exhorted to fight the obesity epidemic, the aim is to win its allegiance for official policies that downplay other issues, like the massive problems of the American health-care system, the continuance of much greater epidemic threats in the world's poor countries, or entrenched differences between the health of the wealthy and that of the poor even within our affluent society. The popularity of the warnings about obesity doesn't hurt the sales of diet products, either.

Like bioterrorism, obesity provides policy makers and profit makers with a justification for managing people's lives and wallets. Also like bioterrorism, the warnings of dire and widespread consequences make obesity suitable as an object of fear. Unlike bioterrorism, though, obesity is no chimera.

Today, Americans, Europeans, and people in many developing countries are heavier than previous generations were. More people are very heavy relative to their height. In this sense, obesity is on the rise and has reached unprecedented levels; if we think that it is a disease, then by the classical epidemiologist's definition it is indeed epidemic.

The World Health Organization calls obesity "one of the greatest public health challenges of the 21st century." According to the U.S. Surgeon General, by 2001 overweight and obesity had become pressing new health challenges, having reached what he called "epidemic proportions" in America. In his introduction to the Surgeon General's report, the scretary of Health and Human Services wrote, "Our modern environment has allowed these conditions to increase at alarming rates and become a growing health problem for our nation. By confronting these conditions, we have tremendous opportunities to prevent the unnecessary disease and disability they portend for our future."

As with bioterrorism, the veracity of the threat obesity represents is impossible to separate from the response to the alleged threat. It isn't even easy to answer the simple question of what obesity is.

Typically, obesity is defined on the basis of the body-mass index (BMI) number. It is calculated by dividing an individual's weight in kilograms by the square of her or his height in meters (in pounds and inches, BMI = weight x 703 / height^2). This measure corrects for the expected increase in weight that accompanies being taller. Today, about 90 percent of Americans have a BMI between 18.5 and 35. People with a BMI between 25 and 29.9 are considered overweight, and those with a BMI of 30 or higher are considered obese. A BMI from 18.5 to 24.9 is medically "normal." By these standards, 34 percent of American adults were obese in 2005–2006, up from 21 percent in 2001. So were between 6 and 27 percent of European adults in recent surveys, varying from country to country.

The BMI cutoffs of 25 and 30, meant to distinguish "healthy" from "unhealthy" weight (i.e., overweight) and "obesity," create a mathematical language by which one size supposedly fits all. A fashion model who is five feet eight (1.73 meters) and weighs 118 pounds (53.6 kilograms) has a BMI of 18. So does a marathoner of the same height and weight. Both are slightly underweight by the common standards, just below "normal." Similarly, both the flabby fifty-year-old businessman who is six feet tall (1.83 m) and weighs 265 pounds (120 kg) and the muscular twenty-one-year-old pro football player of the same height and weight have a BMI of 35. Both are counted as obese. The BMI tells us nothing about fitness. Whether the BMI is the most accurate predictor of illnesses and death supposedly attributable to obesity is open to question (some researchers think waist circumference is a better measure), but all definitions in common use are based on a set of simple physical measurements made on the individual.

It might seem useless to compare an overweight businessman or an underweight model with a professional athlete, but that is only one problem with the BMI standard. Body fatness is self-evidently a continuous spectrum: a few people are extremely thin (models and marathoners, for instance), some are very thin, more are just slim, a great many are medium, a few are slightly fuller than medium-sized, and so forth. But the BMI cutoff turns this continuum of body mass into an either-or. Obesity is like an infection: you have it or you don't. It becomes possible to discriminate who is obese, to distinguish fat people from everyone else with a simple measurement, as we do with tests for HIV infection, or genital herpes, or hepatitis C.

Bad things will happen to the obese individual, according to the CDC and the WHO: diabetes, hypertension, heart disease, stroke, endometrial and breast cancer, gall bladder disease, osteoarthritis, and the metabolic syndrome. Some public-health commentators even refer to an "obesity-diabetes epidemic." The illnesses for which an obese person is allegedly at risk are referred to collectively as "adverse health consequences of obesity," which grants them a cloak of inevitability—although it is clear that most people with a BMI above 30 do not suffer life-threatening illness as a result. A careful review of the studies purporting to show that obesity causes cardiovascular and other diseases found that, apart from osteoarthritis (high body mass has mechanical effects on joints) and estrogen-related cancers (affected by the amount of fat tissue), other illnesses do not show any clear cause-and-effect relation to high body mass.

It is true that obesity can lead to medical problems. But the actual level of body mass at which it becomes likely that physiology will break down and life become short generally lies far above the conventional cutoff line at a BMI of 30. The chances of dying from the effects of obesity are slim enough that the great majority of people who are considered obese by current standards will suffer no shortening of life because of it.

In fact, the obesity epidemic amounts to a far smaller number of deaths than the hype about it would suggest. According to a careful study of U.S. mortality published recently, about 112,000 American deaths in the year 2000 could be attributed to obesity (BMI ≥ 30), roughly 5 percent of all U.S. fatalities. A large-population epidemiologic study cannot rule out contributing causes of death of all sorts, so the true number of obesity-provoked deaths is probably smaller.

The pattern of dying from the obesity epidemic and the extent to which obesity can be said to be the cause of death provokes some questions. Almost all of the excess deaths attributed to obesity occur among people in their sixties (after age sixty-nine obesity has no impact on mortality rates). The mortality among people with high BMI appears to be accounted for largely by incomplete management of diabetes and/or hypertension, two of the main adverse accompaniments of high BMI. Some, and possibly a great many, of the deaths attributed to body mass might equally have been attributed to America's messy health-care system. The good news is that, even with the high cost of medical care in the United States, the impact of body mass on mortality among Americans has been on the decline since 1970. This likely reflects improving medical management of diabetes and hypertension. High BMI is less and less likely to invite early death.

The question of whether obesity can really be said to cause death is further complicated by the labyrinthine pathways by which obesity purportedly connects to disease. Those pathways are affected by hard-to-disentangle factors such as weight cycling (the up-and-down effect of repeated dieting and weight gain), fitness, and use of medications including weight-loss drugs such as Fen-Phen and ephedra, which are themselves linked to cardiovascular problems. The effect of smoking further confounds attempts to link weight to mortality, because smoking, which carries well-known dangers of its own, can be used as a means of weight control. In sum, exactly what the obese person is at risk for is fuzzy, variable, and sometimes not exactly a disease but another risk-conferring condition.

Perhaps it is not surprising, then, that epidemiologic studies of body size and longevity have found that obesity is not particularly deadly. Indeed, people who are overweight by the BMI standard have the lowest mortality rates, even lower than people of "normal" weight. Among adults in their sixties, the age range at which the obesity epidemic supposedly takes the greatest toll, it is far worse to be underweight (BMI < 18.5) than obese. Those with an "obese" BMI of between 30 and 35 have a death rate almost identical to the "normal" BMI group (the rate for the obese is slightly higher but statistically indistinguishable). For Americans in their seventies, the effect of obesity is even less, and the overweight live longest. Even for young people, high BMI is only associated with substantially elevated risk of dying at the very obese BMIs of 35 or more. In effect, longevity is greatest for people who are considered overweight by current medical standards. High body mass has little impact on longevity except for people who are young and even then only at extremely high BMIs. Underweight is the most dangerous body condition of all.

OBESITY AS FALL GUY FOR MODERN FEARS

With the claim that obesity compromises longevity so shaky, it is hard to account for the cries that we are experiencing a dangerous obesity epidemic unless we consider it as a matter of management. Obesity is the fall guy. High body mass itself does not directly cause medically unavoidable death in great numbers. It only causes large numbers of deaths if we are willing to ignore, in the cause-and-effect equation, the failures of the medical care system. The physical suffering of obesity is remediable: obesity crusaders make the advent of "husky" car seats for small children and extra-extra-large clothing sizes sound like cultural catastrophes, but really these are adaptations to increasing size, not harms in themselves. It is the implication of obesity that allows it to be set up as the epidemic at which to direct our fear. It is the sense we get from obesity that we have done something wrong, a sense that is impossible to dodge because of obesity's visibility. With syphilis and AIDS, the invisibility of the dreaded germ and the impossibility of identifying exactly who might be a carrier allowed the imagination to heap presumed carriers with suspicions that derived from racial prejudices and social antipathies. With obesity, its hypervisibility horrifies.

When obesity is said to be an epidemic that threatens the public's health, the meaning of "epidemic" is rejiggered to take advantage of our horror at obesity and its capacity to accommodate our deep-seated fears. The epidemic disease, which is not an illness at all but a condition capable of leading to illness (diabetes, cardiovascular disease, and the so-called metabolic syndrome), is said to cause suffering (low self-esteem, poor school performance) and early death. Obesity's presence is observable to all—it is more effective than the alleged bioterrorist in that way, whose existence the public had to take on faith. Its capacity to produce mayhem isn't apparent, but as with bioterrorism, it can easily take on preexisting fears of destruction. And like the AIDS epidemic, the dangerous thing about obesity is risk—both the risk of adverse consequences and the "risky behavior" that is said to cause it.

In a way, obesity is an epidemic of risk more than it is an epidemic of disease (which it isn't) or death. The risk in question is a tragedy of proportion, literally. Whereas we coded AIDS as a tragedy of excessive appetite in the form of immoderate sexual desire, we regard obesity as a tragedy of appetite for food. The obesity epidemic validates the fearful suspicion that we have let ourselves be seduced by modernity's cornucopia. We eat too much or we eat wrong.

Perhaps disgust is the deepest of the chords by which obesity is defined as an epidemic disease. The disgust elicited by the disfigurement of AIDS victims early on, or by the suppurating wounds that are features of the pretend victims in Atlantic Storm and other biosecurity exercises, gets transposed from the fearsome epidemic disease (AIDS, anthrax, smallpox) onto the dreadful epidemic condition (obesity). Perhaps we are as disgusted by obesity as we were horrified by AIDS or terrified by the prospect of foreign operatives spraying smallpox in the subways. If it is disgust at excessive flesh that helps obesity register as a disease, if risk that helps obesity register as a source of suspicion, then obesity might be the quintessential epidemic in an age in which cause and effect are poorly defined.

With risk in mind and an intent to frame obesity as the thing the public should fear, public health professionals and policy makers are eager to show that the obese person carries risk not only to himself but to others. Some have begun to talk about obesity as a kind of contagion. In 2005 the CDC sent one of its infectious-disease investigation teams to study an "outbreak" of obesity in West Virginia, as if it were SARS or a new type of flu. More recently, an article in a prestigious medical journal reported on research findings showing that obesity can "spread through social networks." Fat people, this sort of reasoning suggests, make their friends fat.

—⁂—

A major component of obesity's fearsome grip on our imaginations today is that it signals poverty. When we say that one reason to be concerned about obesity is that it "affects all segments of society," we don't mean it. Virtually all studies that examine the question in developed countries find that obesity, however defined, is more common among the poor. Once, plumpness signaled wealth. Now, the rich are sleek. In a U.S. national survey, 27 percent of adults who had not finished high school were obese, compared with only 21 percent of adults who had finished college. Poor states, such as Mississippi and Louisiana, have higher prevalences of obesity (26 percent and 23 percent, respectively) than wealthy states, like Connecticut (17 percent). In America, dark skin is associated with obesity, too: In 2001, 31 percent of black adults but only 20 percent of whites reported a BMI of 30 or above. In data from 2006, 53 percent of African American women ages forty to fifty-nine were obese compared with only 39 percent of non-Hispanic white women in that age group. Among women ages sixty or older, the disparity was even greater.

As heaviness is implicitly connected with poverty and powerlessness, the obesity epidemic is a way of telling in new terms the old story: the lower classes or the disdained races threaten the social order. As we become more tolerant of fat people, as we build furniture (and car seats) bigger and cut clothing looser to accommodate larger bodies, as they "infect" others with their size, everyone seems more likely to get fat. We read obesity as a signal that society is on the downgrade.

Associating fatness with powerlessness offers an unfortunate self-fulfilling prophecy. Fat people are the objects of discrimination. They are browbeaten into surgery, ridiculed and humiliated, and in some cases denied employment. In the subliminal equation of body size with powerlessness, an affluent woman who gets fat is slumming, lowering the standards we expect her to observe. Her physician will tell her to do something about her weight, will recommend diet and exercise and, if that doesn't work, medical intervention. If asked about his logic, the doctor will explain he wants his patient to avoid the "inevitable" complications of metabolic syndrome and early death, although these are far from inevitable. Fatness among the affluent and powerful is wrong or "inappropriate." It threatens social collapse.

Recognizing the connection of fatness to powerlessness helps to understand the rhetoric behind fears of obesity. The Surgeon General's 2001 report asserted that although "many people believe that dealing with overweight and obesity is a personal responsibility . . . it is also a community responsibility." Like the English Privy Council's orders of 1543, placing responsibility for plague on "negligence, disorder, and want of charity," the Surgeon General signals that it will be up to citizens to avoid obesity. As parish officials were charged with cleaning up local streets and maintaining plague victims in pesthouses, communities will have to take charge of the obesity crisis. Top-down policy has created national programs on food marketing and advertising and physical activity for schoolchildren in some Western European countries. In the U.S. government's view, as evident in the CDC's "Social-Ecological Model" of obesity, society is an agglomeration of communities; all individuals and their entire private lives, including group activities and bonds of family, friendship, or love, are subsumed within them. The community is expected to deal with the obesity crisis by influencing individuals' "long-term, healthful lifestyle choices." Therefore, national policy on the obesity epidemic remains community-based. A $75 million program of federal grants helps local school boards purchase physical-activity equipment and expand physical education classes, while foundations have donated hundreds of millions of dollars to local obesity-prevention programs. The sense, communicated perfectly by the Surgeon General, is that obesity arises from individuals' errors, but the groups to which those individuals belong must take responsibility.

Aspects of this American approach to obesity are key to understanding the new view of epidemics. Community is supposed to be a defining feature of American social life. Since community is often understood to mean identity group—the African American community, the gay community, the disabled community, and so forth—the U.S. approach lays the blame at the feet of specific groups and avoids associating obesity with any broad social or economic determinants of how people eat or look, or how fat they get. Obesity is depicted as the fault of individuals' poor choices, the failure to opt for the healthy lifestyle. Framed as such, obesity is an easy canvas on which to paint our psychic unease, our difficulties in achieving personal goals, or our sense that we have become lazy—even though no study on the topic of body mass and psychic impairment shows any clear connection.

The obesity epidemic defined as a failure of healthy lifestyle choices makes us attend to how and what we eat. This is perhaps the greatest benefit of the panic over obesity. As a crisis of lifestyle choices, obesity might encourage us to consider the financial profitability or the costs of a food culture that involves extensive processing—a point that is made by the Institute of Medicine of the U.S. National Academy of Sciences. Yet official policies refuse to acknowledge that such factors are actually causes.

By defining obesity as an epidemic of risky eating behavior and as a failure of communities to make healthy choices, policy makers and the corporations they support lead us to lose sight of the structure of modern work: the long hours, the need of hourly wage laborers to hold down two or three different jobs because of the difficulty of landing full-time jobs (employers might then have to pay for health insurance or other benefits), the organization of urban-suburban living arrangements and the consequent need for poorer people to travel further to work, and the unavailability of affordable day care that would allow working mothers some time to shop and cook for their families or to exercise. When we see obesity as an epidemic of unhealthy lifestyle choices, we are not moved to examine the weight-loss industry's interest in perpetuating an ideal of body proportions that is much thinner than the empirically healthiest body size. It makes sure that we will not recognize that the same scientific advisers who claim that obesity is an epidemic crisis are part of a vast research establishment whose funding is entirely dependent on the notion that obesity is a matter of the proper diet or the right amount of exercise.

Obesity is defined as it is in order to manage our focus. The story of the obesity epidemic as told to us is not about a system responsible for making our waistlines grow but about demons *within* the system—social faults, failures of community, bad relationships, and more. These demons are dangerous to us all, and obesity is the sign of the danger, a symptom of the devilry of inappropriate lifestyle choices. Like the epidemic infections of syphilis, polio, or AIDS, obesity is the deserved result of imprudence, injudicious choices, or inability to control one's appetite. The obesity epidemic embodies a number of stories. It is a tale of how bad habits threaten social stability, how quickly danger can spread (with obesity playing the part of an infection), how risky life is, and how much our society has declined from an imagined era of healthier choices (the "good old days"). The obesity epidemic expresses both our misgivings about how we lead our lives today and our unceasing fascination with how we look.

MANAGING MISGIVINGS ABOUT PARENTING: CHILDHOOD OBESITY

The strongest language about epidemic obesity seems to come out when we talk about children. Childhood obesity is an American national catastrophe, according to the acting Surgeon General. The president of the Robert Wood Johnson Foundation warns that "these kids" might incur inescapable and "corrosive" costs to their health and well-being. Saying "these kids" gestures to them collectively, as if they were an ethnic group or a nationality. The epidemic "robs them of their childhood," says a university health researcher. A CDC official likens obesity to a "wave that is just moving through the population." Tragic sentiment prevails.

The American Public Health Association, calling overweight the "biggest problem facing children today," asserts that the crisis is increasing because of children's inactivity and poor eating habits. But since children can hardly be held wholly responsible, the fault implicitly lies with their parents and their schools. "Inactivity and poor eating habits" means that Americans are doing a poor job at rearing and schooling their children. The APHA does recognize the deep roots of the problem, which are entangled in international and national economic policies, the structure of the health-care and education systems, community organization, and other aspects of the institutions of American life. But however complex the root system of this "hidden epidemic," the APHA attributes childhood obesity to "too much food and too little exercise."

The obesity epidemic is shaping a modern Progressive movement. Beyond food and exercise, the APHA asserts that the basic problem behind childhood obesity includes lack of "quality time" with parents, the increase in divorce, the "latchkey phenomenon," and a "barrage of images and ideas" from the media and television. The APHA, a large, redoubtable, and usually liberal-minded organization of health professionals, turns to social conservatives' code words to explain the obesity crisis. With "latchkey" it alludes to the dangers of women entering the workforce. It points to divorce as a key ingredient of the social crisis of childhood obesity. It condemns *ideas*. With childhood obesity, public-health professionals make common cause with America's most moralistic factions. The first movement of Progressives, a century ago, united medicine and moralism, attacking the sexual activities it found morally reprobate (adultery, prostitution) under the mantle of social hygiene. This time around, overeating and laziness bother the Progressives. Healthy eating and physical activity in the fight against childhood obesity are the new social hygiene.

In the Progressive view, childhood obesity reveals the culture's essential flaw. As with the sexual hygiene Progressivism promoted a century ago, the mechanics by which the flaw turns into a social problem are a little hazy. In those days it was divorce, industrialization, urbanization, and women joining the workforce and finding a political voice. Today, women joining the workforce, television and the Internet, and exposure to images and ideas are understood as contributing factors to the latest social disgrace.

—⁂—

The epidemic of childhood obesity reworks facts to suit the story. The data available do show an increase over the past few years in the proportion of U.S. children who are overweight (about 17 percent of adolescent Americans now are considered overweight according to the National Center for Health Statistics, compared to about 11 percent circa 1990 and only 5 percent in the late 1970s, and the proportion of overweight children is also increasing in Europe). But the rhetoric of the epidemic tends to obscure meaning. For instance, when a private group concerned with childhood obesity analyzed the U.S. data, it found 35 percent of school-age children to be overweight—twice the prevalence noted by the federal agency.

The major problem in interpreting findings on the rise of overweight or obesity among children is the sleight of hand used in managing the statistics. Part of the reworking of facts involves the definition of obesity itself—the meaning of the term is no less elusive for children than for adults, but for children it is also fraught with emotional overlay. There is no consensus on the BMI indicating obesity in a child. Therefore, the more inclusive term "overweight" is used instead, and sometimes "obesity" and "overweight" are used interchangeably.

Even the standards for overweight in children are shaky. The usual method for diagnosing overweight in a child is to compare the child's weight to the distribution of weights of 1960s- and '70s-era children at the same height and age, standardized to the 1977 population. Since there is no standard for obesity in a child, a statistical trick is performed: health professionals will say that a child is obese if he or she is above the ninety-fifth percentile of the weight-for-height distribution at the same age in 1977. This is a little bit like claiming that innate intelligence is improving because a higher proportion of today's high schoolers score in what used to be the upper 5 percent of the IQ distribution compared to kids of a generation ago.

The alarm about childhood obesity twists the postmodern epidemic into a self-defining loop. The problem with childhood obesity is that fat children are more likely to become fat adults. The problem with fat adults is that they are more likely to develop certain metabolic and physiologic problems, such as diabetes. Although it can be costly to treat these problems, they are not immediately or often deadly. Since the possibility of illness or early death makes us define excess weight in an adult as risky, the possibility of becoming an extremely fat adult thereby makes being an extremely fat child risky, and the possibility of producing an extremely fat child obligates us to prevent *any* extra weight in a child.

With risk looming, allowing a child to become fat becomes a harmful act. And because obesity is a global crisis or simply because the costs of treating the possible consequences of excess weight, like diabetes, can be high, allowing a child to get fat is considered a kind of civic misdeed, too. It must be avoided in itself, even if there are no immediate adverse consequences. Anything that would make a child fat is tainted, no matter how unlikely to lead to weight gain. Divorce. Television. Ideas. Childhood obesity is like sexual predation or satanic ritual abuse—we can use it as a rationale for decrying elements of the culture that seem immoral and for vilifying, ostracizing, and in some cases indicting the people who embrace them. In short order, all of childhood seems to be a risky endeavor, filled with danger for the society. The childhood obesity epidemic contributes to the broader impulse toward refashioning childhood itself as a period of both intense vulnerability and grave toxicity to society—despite the lack of evidence of widespread harm. The perception of childhood's riskiness is evident in the hysteria over Internet predators, concern over kids' exposure to images of smokers on TV and in movies, parental warnings on music and video games, and other panics.

One manifestation of seeing childhood obesity as an epidemic of risk is that we create administrative solutions to manage our children's behavior. If necessary, programs will even force kids to act right. If childhood obesity is the threat that it seems to be, then we feel justified in demanding that government programs manage our children. It starts to seem right to us that the government should help kids avoid the criminal elements that would fatten them, and guide them toward the correct (thin) path. The "We Can!" and "Media-Smart Youth: Eat, Think and Be Active" anti-obesity programs of the National Institute on Child Health and Human Development and federal programs on "Youth Risk Behavior," "Key Strategies to Prevent Obesity," and "Food-Safe Schools" imply that improper diet is not merely a threat to the well-being of some children but pathological among America's kids in general. Behaviorally oriented programs like these give form to the powerful social message that eating is a threat. The management of diet, along prescribed lines, is thus a public responsibility.

To call childhood obesity an epidemic is to resurrect "epidemic" in its earliest sense. This epidemic is native. It is home—and not only in the sense that largeness seems to be characteristic of modern postindustrial societies but also in that it has to do with what happens in our homes. The terms we use to speak of the epidemic of childhood obesity implicate our own child rearing. The childhood obesity epidemic raises a warning finger at how we create, conduct, and end our marriages, and laments the decline of home cooking, the rise of the restaurant meal, the popularity of the snack meal, the solitary meal, or the on-the-go meal. These facets of the culture take on a moral tone and civic import. We reveal an anxiety that there is something wrong with our culture and our relationships. This need to define a new problem in society is reminiscent of responses to epidemics past. Unlike earlier epidemics, though, childhood obesity is not merely about groups of people we don't like because of their skin color or allegedly reprobate behavior, nor is it about a threat allegedly lurking inside technical innovations. It points to a flaw in society. Childhood obesity signals that our society has broken with tradition. We have deviated from the traditional family structure and gender roles and work arrangements and, most of all, eating habits.

The obesity epidemic reminds us that, in a society geared for success, to look different and fail to achieve what is expected is to be both abnormal and frightening. We no longer put to death the carriers of threat to the social order. Instead, we diagnose the different. We declare them risky. Readily enough, we equate riskiness with untoward happenstances: HIV infection becomes identical with AIDS, hypertension with heart disease, obesity with diabetes. The disease melds with its premonitory signs (no matter that the premonitory sign might point only faintly to the dreadful outcome). And the signs are tightly linked with behaviors that supposedly give rise to them. We pathologize danger.

AUTISM, THE ADMINISTRATIVE EPIDEMIC

Obesity's counterweight is the autism epidemic. Like the obese in a culture that adores thinness, autistic people are out of place in a culture favoring flexibility, rapidity, and multiplicity of communication. And the autistic child's difficulties in school command attention in a society in which poor school performance is understood to signal low earning potential. Like obesity, autistic behavior demands a diagnosis. Also like obesity, autism is supposedly newly epidemic—and therefore the autism epidemic can be taken to signal new failures.

Autism does not have obesity's hypervisibility, and autistic children are not accused of harboring future hazard or spreading risk. But autism readily highlights our fears about the adequacy of our parenting as well as anxiety about the future of our productive society.

Autism is a condition of mind that is managed as a psychiatric disorder. In fact, autistic ways of living in the world are so broad and variable that psychiatrists have created a whole set of diagnoses to accommodate the many forms of autistic difference: the so-called autism spectrum disorders. The ASD include classic autism, Asperger's syndrome, pervasive developmental disorder, and childhood disintegrative disorder, plus the genetically determined Rett's disorder. All are characterized by particular limitations of social interaction, attention, and communication, often with repetitive behavior and sometimes with difficulties in language learning.

Autism occurs in about 0.6 percent of children in the United States and Europe, about one child out of every 160. It begins early in childhood, never after age three. Although evidence in historical documents suggests that autistic individuals have been noticed for centuries, autism was not recognized as a psychiatric problem before the early 1900s, when psychiatrists' attention to children veered away from the effort to keep them out of asylums and toward identifying the roots of socially aberrant behavior. The autism spectrum, which seemed to be marked by disengagement, was then considered a behavioral aspect of mental illness: the adjective "autistic" was coined in 1912 by a Swiss psychiatrist as a description of symptoms shown by certain children who were considered schizophrenic. Autism and Asperger's syndrome, the first two main specifiable autistic conditions, were identified as distinct psychiatric problems in the 1940s. Autism did not appear in the *Diagnostic and Statistical Manual of Mental Disorders*, the American Psychiatric Association's gold standard for diagnosis, until 1980, as a subcategory of childhood schizophrenia. The ASD appears in the most recent revision of the *DSM* (1994) as a distinct set of diagnoses.

The particularizing of autistic behavior as mental disorder owes much to modern anxieties about childhood. It is intrinsically part of the importance we give to education as an emblem of success and the pathologizing of failure in a society whose social order demands achievement. Certainly, the establishment of autism is intertwined with the developing role of psychiatry as a preventive of social instability.

The alacrity with which our society has written the epidemic tale about autism is revealing. Perhaps autistic styles resonate for us as disorders nowadays because, like the bodily style of obesity, they seem to embody the very processes of contemporary life that we find most troubling. The autistic child is said to be disengaged emotionally, and emotional disengagement is supposedly characteristic of contemporary social interaction—we bowl alone; our social ties are numbed, allegedly abetted by the Internet and the mobile phone; we play at personal computer games in isolation. The autistic child pays uncanny attention to detail and might recite data repeatedly and fondly, much as our reliance on statistics and lists allegedly makes modern life superficial and saps us of deep humanistic involvement. The autistic child's attention span can be minuscule, and limited attention span is typical of the modern multitasker who supposedly misses out on authentic experience. The autistic style, being different from what we expect yet reminding us of what we revile in modernity, becomes a pathology.

—✳—

Autism is the postmodern epidemic of nothing. Autistic behavior is not dangerous in itself nor is it very uncommon—it is just difference transformed into disease by the way we talk about it.

To claim, as many do, that more children are born autistic today than ever before is to make an assertion no data can support. Before autism was defined as a psychiatric condition, there was no information about its prevalence. As the understanding of what autism means has changed, so have diagnostic standards. The prevalence measured in earlier eras cannot be compared with that of today. To claim that autism occurs more often now is to express anxieties about the thinking-and-feeling demands of contemporary life by inventing a disease, diagnosing it widely, and construing its ubiquity as an objective threat—as grounds for well-justified fear rather than troubling anxiety. To talk about autism as an epidemic is also to appoint psychiatrists as surrogate watchers, much as the obesity epidemic has empowered physicians, nutritionists, and health educators to define a threat in fatness and tell us what to do about it.

Is autism more common now? Undoubtedly it is—because we recognize and diagnose it. The increase in prevalence of autism is administrative: it is revealed through an increased awareness of autism, earlier diagnosis (which expands the total number of people who have ever been diagnosed with it), rediagnosis as autism of what used to be called schizophrenia, and the expansion of autism to encompass related conditions (that is, creating the ASD). Now people with an ASD diagnosis represent a larger proportion of the population than in the past, even as recently as the 1980s. Leo Kanner, the psychiatrist who first declared autism to be a distinct condition of children in 1943, estimated that it occurred in about 3 children out of every 10,000 in that era; studies from the mid-1960s through the early 1990s estimated prevalence on average at around 4.7 per 10,000; and current estimates are 13 per 10,000 for autism alone and about 60 per 10,000 for the entire ASD (which is equal to the one-in-160 figure). That means ASD now looks to be about twentyfold more common than Kanner's 1940s estimate.

To psychiatrists and psychologists who see autism as one outcome of central-nervous-system development in early childhood, probably genetically determined, the expansion of autism prevalence was predictable. By the 1990s they knew that it would become more widely recognized and that it would be more likely to be diagnosed, since special programs for autistic children would become more effective and available. And that is exactly what has happened.

The largest part of the increase in ASD prevalence over the past generation has been in the diagnostic categories of severest impairment and most minimal impairment—the two extremes of the spectrum. The former group likely represents children who were formerly diagnosed as mentally retarded; the latter would include many children who once received no diagnosis at all. The newest diagnoses, childhood disintegrative disorder and Asperger's syndrome, both added to the DSM in 1994, now comprise three-quarters of new ASD diagnoses. These details of the pattern of the expanding autism epidemic suggest that much of the increase in autism's presence in our society comes from diagnostic practice.

Psychiatry is not the sole moving force in shaping an autism epidemic, though. Our society has collaborated in defining the autistic style as reflecting a disordered psyche. We seem to want it to be a disease. We can hear this in the dialogue about autism, with its grammar drawn from the germ-theory model of causation. Because we encounter autistic children more commonly now than before, and because the autistic mode is now a psychiatric diagnosis, people who are discontent with the customary neurodevelopmental explanation for the condition seek a germlike causal explanation for what appears to be a disease outbreak. Difference, diagnosed, turns our attention to dangerous "germs."

In particular, many people have fixed blame on state policies for what they allege (erroneously) to be a new epidemic of autism. They single out vaccination programs. In their view, government's attempt to protect us from nature by applying technology to create vaccines also creates new threats. In the United States, the anti-vaccination movement usually fixes on thimerosal (called thiomersal in Europe), an organomercury compound once used as a preservative in vaccines. In Britain, it has focused on the MMR (measles-mumps-rubella) immunization.

For the antivaccinationists, it isn't foreigners or suspicious immigrants who are suspect in the autism epidemic; it's the government. Alleging that vaccines induce autism is a way of trying to make sense of the increasing commonness of ASD by fixing on an expanding danger in the environment, a danger created by government plans. In part, this is an old story: people have read into epidemics their fears about government power, loss of liberty, and the perils of technological advance at least since the plague outbreaks of the 1600s. But the allegations that our children's minds are being disordered through state policy resonate with modern suspicions of big business, big government, or Big Pharma ruining the environment we live in or the health of our children.

To accept the explanation that the autism epidemic is an administrative artifact of how we seek out, find, and diagnose the condition rather than an untoward effect of government policies would undercut the basis for the vaccine accusations. For people who suspect that their government had a hand in their children's autism, the anti-immunization uprising expresses their disappointment and fright and transforms them into a fear of toxic vaccines. Framing the autism epidemic as a matter of dangerous technology, nefarious vaccine manufacturers, or lax government oversight converts the fright of having autistic children into someone else's responsibility.

Autism doesn't spread. Since it begins only in childhood, those adults who are not already autistic are not going to become autistic. But we experience surprise and concern when we find ourselves having to interact with or rear so many autistic children. Attributing this discomfiture to a larger and more pernicious conspiracy turns the fright into fear (what *else* are these companies putting into our children? should I stop using all pediatric medications?) and anxiety (what yet-unknown harms will we discover as time goes on?).

A 2005 essay by Robert F. Kennedy Jr. called "Deadly Immunity" provided substantial driving force to the U.S. antivaccination movement. The article offers an account of a CDC conference in 2000 in which the information that thimerosal causes autism was, according to Kennedy, quashed. He writes, "The story of how government health agencies colluded with Big Pharma to hide the risks of thimerosal from the public is a chilling case study of institutional arrogance, power and greed." But corruption is not causation. It is easy to demonstrate that thimerosal does not cause autism. Thimerosal was no longer used in vaccine preparations given routinely to U.S. children after 2001, and even by a conservative estimate, American children have not been exposed to mercury through vaccination for well over five years. If thimerosal were a cause of autism, there would have been a sharp drop in diagnoses beginning in 2005 or 2006. But no such decline has occurred.

Other theories offering different explanations for epidemic autism also attract people who are disappointed with the conventional view or distrustful of mainstream science. British physician Andrew Wakefield and his colleagues proposed that a "leaky gut" allows toxins, presumed to be more abundant in the modern environment, access to the developing child's nervous system. The leaky-gut group specifically cast suspicion on the MMR vaccine, which seemed to be linked temporally to the onset of autism in some children.

The Kennedy article, the Wakefield theory, and numerous books and articles by others bearing on the thimerosal theory or the MMR theory all contain the right ingredients to reassure the anxious that they are right to be worried. There are the profit-hungry pharmaceutical companies, there is the collaboration between government and industry, there is the official cover-up. And there is danger lurking in the environment, specifically in the man-made environment of modernity. The central theme of the emerging-infections era, "danger hidden within," asserts itself in the theories of autism's causation.

The real problem isn't whether vaccination, a leaky gut, some specific component of certain vaccines, or another danger newly abundant in the modern environment causes autism. It is not that autism is truly spreading in the fashion of traditional contagion. The problem is that the controversy over causes makes autism seem less like a broad spectrum of normative mental-emotional states and more like an illness. As with other postmodern epidemics, the dialogue about the nature and origin of the epidemic helps create the epidemic.

When theories about autism's basis seem to invoke the emerging-infections narrative—that is, that danger lurks in our modern arrangements (in this case, immunizations)—the creators of the emerging-infections account hasten to correct them. Instead of responding by saying autism is not a disorder, so it need not have a cause, they hold only that there is no evidence that autism is caused by vaccines. In so doing, they seem to confirm the assertion that autism is a disease and does have a cause. This makes it look even more like an epidemic, not just a rise in prevalence resulting from administrative changes.

—⁂—

Without the twentieth-century transformation of psychiatry into an instrument of public health—what some call the "mental hygiene" movement—autism could not be an epidemic today. It took a half-century after the "discovery" of autism by psychiatrists before it was classified as a distinct disorder and became accessible to the epidemic story. Although there was an evolution in thinking about autism, a dramatic change was precipitated by a new focus on schools and teachers. When the obesity epidemic returned risk to the home, it generated health-backed expectations of how we will conduct our private lives (less fat, more whole grains, no latchkey kids!). The autism epidemic delegates responsibility for dealing with children's behavior to the schools, and that has led schools to create more programs, which has led to more diagnosis.

Why school success is a desirable commodity in today's society is complicated, and perhaps inscrutable. But self-evidently, success in school translates into opportunities for higher education and career. We value schools today over and above whatever value we place on learning: we expect them to be institutions of ethics education, administering the lessons that deliver modern middle-class mores; we assume they will be organs of acculturation, providing early lessons in civics and "conflict resolution"; and we want them to be therapeutic, making it possible for the less able to succeed. Naturally, children whose social engagement is limited or different, who communicate less, or who integrate language slowly—children who behave autistically, that is—do less well. It is no longer acceptable to place such children in asylums. We expect that the social-ethical-therapeutic modes of school will be available even to them. It was necessary, therefore, to make it possible for schools to accommodate the autistic.

The autism epidemic's interface with schooling explains, in part, why autism sounds so loud in the contemporary social dialogue. School success, like thinness, is an expectation of the middle classes in today's society. To be unable to succeed in school is another mark of powerlessness. As with obesity, so the autism epidemic has created incentives for the affluent to devote money and resources to treating what has now been diagnosed as a disorder—and in some cases to demand that treatment services be extended to the poor, too. This aligning of services for the diagnosed with wherewithal, and with the politics of social justice, helps to consolidate the epidemic story.

In the United States, the Individuals with Disabilities Education Act (IDEA), passed by Congress in 1990, brought autism and school systems into a semblance of concord. IDEA requires that American public-school districts offer individualized educational programs to students with recognized disabilities, autism included, and provides for incentive funding to states. School districts accordingly established accommodations, including special classes, tutoring, and other programs, for children with autism diagnoses. Autism was recognized as a legitimate qualification for IDEA by the Department of Education beginning with the 1991–1992 school year. This change made a big difference to parents of "difficult" children or those with "discipline problems." If their children are diagnosed with an ASD, they become eligible for more attention from the educational system. IDEA also created a rationale for psychiatrists' response to autistic children, expanding the criteria for diagnosis and liberalizing diagnostic practice (e.g., earlier diagnosis).

After IDEA, with its incentives for diagnosis, autism quickly became more common. In the fourteen school years between 1992–1993 and 2005–2006, the Department of Education reported a twelvefold increase in the number of students with ASD diagnoses; among adolescents in particular, the increase was about sixteenfold.

Diagnosis has a double edge. It is a way of marking threat and allowing for it to be managed. But it is also a way of providing greater access. In a society dedicated to the myth that dreams are shared and that we all have access to the same dream fulfillments (we all, supposedly, want the good job and the large house in the suburbs), diagnosis is an important way to assure that opportunities are afforded. The autism epidemic is a way of expanding opportunities. The cost is that it makes autism a disorder.

The new awareness of ASD as a mental disorder misreads what is largely just a different way of being as if it were an illness. In the long run, the extensive diagnosis, intense and special attention to the problem, and even the sometimes-irrational arguments over the causes of autism might contribute to better acceptance of difference. In this hopeful view, the present uproar over autism might be the birth trauma of a new awareness. But the controversy over autism offers a window onto how powerful the epidemic is as a narrative— how useful it can be, and how little need it has for genuine illness as its basis.

—〰—

The postmodern epidemic is a crisis not because illness is spreading or indiscriminate death looms. It is a crisis because the powerful deem it to be such. As obesity reminds us, an epidemic can now be a matter of management—managing the public's fear of social disintegration and untimely death by providing an object on which we can project our dread, managing anxiety about the poor by recoding powerlessness as disease threat, bringing the question of our future health home and making it a matter of how we raise our children or run our households. As autism reminds us, an epidemic can be an administrative effect, the result of laudable attempts to provide for people who seem different and the concomitant popularizing of a problem that was once neglected. An epidemic can take shape when there is a new diagnosis making the different disordered, and when we accommodate their needs and yet project onto their very presence our fears that something has gone wrong. In the contemporary epidemic, our governments have messed too much with nature, or modernity has messed too much with us. The advance of our culture has also left us vulnerable. Something that has lingered among us for a long time suddenly looks both ubiquitous and mortally threatening. Overweight adults and children whose behavior is unusual suddenly become exemplars of the threat of modern life, unprecedented and uniquely dangerous. All of which gives those who have power more reason to wield it and new ways to hold on to it, and gives those who sell us devices and treatments to handle each respective threat more opportunity to profit.

THE RISK-FREE LIFE

To prolong life was not one of Ravelstein's aims.
Risk, limit, death's blackout were present in
every living moment.

—Saul Bellow, *Ravelstein*

L ife is never without risks. That sounds like a self-evident fact,
yet how easily we lose sight of it. For Saul Bellow to say about
his main character, a great lover of good food, drink, and other men,
that risk was to him an acceptable, even celebratory fact of life was
to depict a human of a rare type in the modern world. Unlike Ravelstein, most of us are preoccupied with risk. We will adopt manifold
caution in the service of postponing death's blackout. But the Rav-
elsteins of this world see something most of us have missed. To wish
to escape peril entirely is to yearn for the unattainable. Nobody can
live forever, let alone healthy, blemish-free, and slim. When we talk
about epidemics caused by bioterrorism or obesity, we speak of rampant potentiality, spreading *risk*. We are both seeking relief from
something real and longing for something not at all real: the life
without risk.

The epidemic of risk needs no germ or even a disease. Widespread death is not an essential ingredient. Today's epidemics depend

on a chain of other facts, more elusive ones: a sense of fatal fault, a conviction that there is something wrong with our society, a suspicion that the flaw is spreading some kind of malaise. Uneasy people will be easy to convince that there is something wrong. The epidemic requires no clear idea as to what the malaise is (although a diagnosis is essential) or what causes it. The rhetoric of risk and danger are sufficient to start the epidemic engines.

Nature continues to produce epidemics of real disease. The rising incidence of infection with antibiotic-resistant staph strains, MRSA, is a reminder that even the powerful weapons of the twentieth-century battle with contagion won only temporary victories. Sporadic cases of human disease caused by bird viruses, such as West Nile and avian flu, attest to the continuing capacity for new threats to arise out of the complex interactions of different species. Repeated outbreaks of food-borne illness, like those associated with milk in China and lettuce in the United States, demonstrate that the suspicion that technological advance invites untoward consequences is not pure fantasy. Food-production methods that can make food more abundant may also open the door to potentially dangerous organisms. The epidemic of MRSA, occasional outbreaks of food-associated gastroenteritis, and West Nile attest to a continuing and well-placed concern with the potential for real germs to take us by surprise and cause real epidemic illness.

Yet even in the case of epidemics of real disease, media commentators and the many officials who pander to them together craft the now-customary epidemic story. It is a tale of lurking dangers and hidden risks: hospital errors, food-processing mistakes, disease carriers flying on commercial airline flights, or Americans' penchant for jalapeños in our fast-food burritos will be blamed. The sense will be communicated that the threat lies either in technology or human appetites, or in the way they interact. There will be mention of the lack of oversight—the diminution of food-inspection programs, for instance. There might be mention of real capacities of different bacteria to evolve in directions that are unpredictable and for bacterial populations to bloom inexplicably, aspects of microecology that remain mysterious to us. There will be a note about the impossibility of predicting which viruses will suddenly become pathogenic. But the main story will transmit two take-home messages: the modern world is filled with risk, and the imminent danger is dreadful. The epidemic story today might be removed from the reality of suffering, but it is never far from risk.

THE SENSE OF RISK AND
SUSCEPTIBILITY TO MANIPULATION

The power of our collective sense of risk is most evident in the many, and much-discussed, epidemics whose imaginary germs lurk in our character, our modern psyche, or our technology. Concerns about crystal-meth abuse, road rage, teen suicide, attention-deficit/ hyperactivity disorder (ADHD), binge drinking, and Internet predation are all driven more by a fear that modernity has heightened our vulnerability than by actual statistics showing harm to health or shortened lives. Unlike polio, syphilis, cholera, or any of the genuine disease threats of old, the diagnosis in the new epidemic is not a mark of impending injury or even a stigma identifying the sufferer as a dangerous carrier. Diagnosis is a pointer, directing the victims toward whichever therapeutic entity is supposed to be able to treat the disorder: addiction-treatment services, twelve-step programs, behavior modification, after-school programs, pharmaceutical products (often, pharmaceutical fixes are the point of the diagnosis), and so forth. The existence (and in some cases profitability) of these "interventions" supports the continuing stream of newly diagnosed "victims." The resulting expansion of the prevalence of the condition supports the idea that it is an epidemic. The presence of the epidemic justifies the many structures put in place to deal with it. It's a perfectly vicious circle.

With many of the new epidemics, the origin is not stated. No-body who claims there is an epidemic of crystal-meth abuse or binge drinking will say that it comes from a specific cause. The cause is un-derstood to reside either in a failure of modern life to meet personal needs or in some technical overreach. The triggers for the epidemics of obesity, ADHD, teen suicide, and so forth are assumed to be nox-ious influences residing in the physical or social environment—bad parenting, overexposure to TV, bullying, and the like. These dangers in the contemporary world supposedly make life risky and make us vulnerable. It is easy to believe that vaccines make our kids autistic, our food (or the way we eat it) makes us fat, or the availability of psy-choactive substances makes us addicts. The paradoxical triumph of germ theory makes it no longer necessary to find a germ to be able to assert what caused an epidemic. The cause is presumed to be simple, hidden, and lurking in the way we live.

In the new epidemic story line, the hidden physiology of modern society includes demonic technological advances that seduce us with the come-on of a better life but then interact mysteriously with our appetites to put us in danger. When we feel uncomfortable, when we are hopeless, or when our children are sick, this scenario might be easy to believe. Government officials and opposition ac-tivists proffer advice to keep us out of danger: stay away from televi-sion so as not to become obese, keep vaccines away from our kids so they won't become autistic, forbid minors to buy alcohol so they won't become binge drinkers.

The fear that modernity has created unique and unprecedented vulnerabilities leaves us open to manipulation by people who seek support for their political agendas or moral campaigns. When we send our kids to weight-loss camp, place parental controls on their Internet use, and teach them that abstinence is the only healthy ap-proach to sex until they are married, we think we will not only ben-efit ourselves or our own children but that we will help to stop an epidemic. By declaring a problem to be epidemic, the powerful assert a right to manage it, and in managing it they tell us how we should act.

The epidemic of risk is a real shift both in the history of the epidemic idea and in the management of epidemics by people with power to maintain or something to sell. "Epidemic" came to refer to a disease outbreak only after people threw out the ancient notion of disaster as an expression of nature's fickleness. Calamity became the result of a logical turn of events—the arrow of an angry Apollo or the hand of God. After Hippocrates, epidemic disease could be appreciated as having its own logic, independent of supernatural explanations and seated in observable patterns of the natural world. The epidemic idea thus began as a reflection of humankind's expanding attempts to make sense of the universe. And as much as the narratives of epidemic disease continued to reflect beliefs in divine punishment, as plague came and went, and then cholera, typhus, smallpox, polio, and more, the story of an epidemic increasingly depended on the logic of rational observation.

So it's paradoxical that new epidemic crises depend not on observation at all but on a kind of reading of the auguries, forecasting future harm. The epidemic seems to be returning to a more ancient sensibility, attempting to wrest coherence from an inherently inscrutable universe. The paradox is that the universe is more knowable than ever, and sometimes the very people who are responsible for extending our knowledge of the world—scientists, that is—assist in portraying epidemics as constantly, bewilderingly threatening.

FINANCIAL PANIC AND EPIDEMIC PANIC

Risk was at the core of the 2008 financial disaster, in many accounts. Depending on where one stood, it was the fault of mortgage lenders' mismanagement of risk, home buyers who had overestimated their means, insurers who backed the mortgage lenders, the system of leveraged financial dealings (credit default swaps and so forth) that enabled the insurers to overreach, or the federal government's lack of oversight. Somewhere, there was a failure of risk management.

There is some truth in each of these claims. But the meltdown was a system disaster, complex and unforeseeable if you looked at only one piece of the puzzle, watched only one actor, or studied only one risk. Still, to acknowledge the complexity of such a disaster would be to assert that no single element of risk could be held to account, that no one change would have made the difference between yesterday's boom and the recession that followed the meltdown. Instead, most observers turned their attention to parsing the type and intensity of the risk involved.

We narrate epidemic crises similarly. We portray an epidemic as the result of one failure or another. Almost always, we presume that an epidemic resulted because of the mismanagement of small risks. AIDS is the fault of people not using condoms, we say, or having too many sex partners; obesity is the fault of adults not exercising enough, kids watching too many advertisements for junk food on TV, or the abundance of corn syrup in grocery items; autism is the fault of vaccines. Social conservatives blame our bad habits, while liberals bemoan the lack of governmental oversight. And officials tell us all to "reduce our risk."

Like the recent financial crisis, epidemics are system disasters. Yet here, too, few people will admit as much. To acknowledge that an epidemic is a system disaster would be to acknowledge the emptiness of the behavioral turn. It would be to admit that epidemics are complex, multicausal, and determined more powerfully by interacting forces in the environment—in nature or within our social milieu, just as financial crises occur in the environment of global finance.

The self-amplifying quality of the financial crisis is also reminiscent of epidemic disease. Not, primarily, in the sense of germs spreading fast and wildly—in truth, that's common in movies but doesn't happen very often with real microbes (and when it does happen, it tends to give way fairly quickly to a more indolent pattern of spread).

The panicky transmission of financial insecurity parallels the movement of dread when an epidemic threatens. The way the drop in the housing market triggered instability in the insurance industry, then spread to investment firms, Wall Street, banks, durable-goods producers, and so on reprised the panics that accompanied AIDS and SARS and, nowadays, surrounds obesity. Anyone who remembers the calls to tattoo homosexual men and prohibit gays from teaching school in the 1980s or, more recently, the falloff in patronage at Chinese restaurants in the United States when Americans feared contracting SARS in 2003 knows how contagious panic can be, and how pernicious.

In both sorts of crisis, focusing our attention on minutia of risk—on "toxic assets," unhealthy behavior, unhealthy investment, bad judgment—masks the larger unfathomable complexity from which disasters spring. And in both cases the disaster is fueled by panic over the prospect of disaster itself.

MODERNITY AND DREAD

Dread is key. By claiming to foresee epidemics, crystal-ball gazers play on our fears. Humans have always needed an object on which to displace inchoate fears of the unknown. As society developed and the civilized life provided advantages over the feral one, the solitary one, or the nomadic one, additional fears naturally arose about the potential destruction of ever-more-comfortable society. And as society has now come to control its own future, or to claim that it does, the future threat is as suitable an object for subconscious fears and awakened anxieties as was the present danger of plague five centuries ago.

Modernity can elicit anxieties, in other words. The sociologist Anthony Giddens writes that modernity can "disturb the fixity of things." By creating new pathways by which we are driven to live our lives, it "colonizes a segment of a novel future." Discomfort of this

sort probably has much to do with our feeling that disaster is imminent, even though we live in a society in which disaster is demon-
strably less likely than ever. We mess with nature to make life better,
we're successful at it—life really is better. But maybe we can't help
but worry that we've messed too much. The death and destruction
caused by heat waves in Europe in 2003, Hurricane Katrina in 2005,
and the 2008 earthquake in China remind us that the benefits of
modern technology and institutions can be illusory.

Hidden anxieties about modern life can blind us to just how safe
technology has made our lives. We can afford to tell the epidemic
story about obesity, attention deficit, or crystal meth because we are
very good at controlling contagion nowadays. Although SARS killed
hundreds of people in Asia in 2003, it was brought under control very
quickly. And where there was warning—in the United States, for
instance—SARS outbreaks were completely averted through implementation of simple disease-control precautions. West Nile virus will
be controlled, eventually, using programs that suppress mosquito populations without spraying toxic pesticides, like application of *Bacillus
thuringiensis*, a bacterium that devours mosquito larvae. Polio, once
the scourge of middle-class children, has been eradicated in the
United States through mass vaccination campaigns and one day will
be eradicated from the globe. Smallpox has been eradicated worldwide. Because of improvements in sanitation and changes in the structure of urban society, the last major cholera outbreaks in the United
States or Europe occurred in 1866. Empirically speaking, our world is
far, far safer than that of our grandparents and great-grandparents. But
the gaze of the worried isn't fixed on all the evidence. Anxiety is no
statistician.

In one sense, the capacity to collect more and more data about
how the world works might itself be a cause of anxiety. The very
prominence of epidemics like obesity and potential epidemics like
avian flu in media reports and, therefore, given our media-soaked culture, throughout contemporary discussion makes it easier to imagine

that something is amiss. The incessant exhortation to worry issued by officials, backed by scientific findings, and amplified by media makes the public more susceptible to anxiety and more easily manipulated.

Officials who have a program that will make them look aggressive in combating risk and corporations that have something to sell create worry about epidemic threats. A public that suspects that destruction impends can then believe that redemption is still available. In response to today's epidemics of obesity, binge drinking, and so forth, there are online health-educational modules that will alert us to how risky our lives are and therapeutic programs that will supposedly limit the damage. Advocacy groups urge legislators to pass laws that will, they claim, limit these threats. All of this management of new epidemics urges on the public a new kind of piety, in which everyone is supposed to worship at the altar of "healthy lifestyle choices." Our leaders conduct the biopreparedness exercises to redeem us from the grip of the evil. Others demand of Hollywood that only the bad guys in movies smoke cigarettes. Magazines advertise diet plans; federal agencies tell us to talk to our children about drugs. Our health professionals and policy makers deliver the sort of moral messages that, not long ago, were given only by pastors in their Sunday sermons. Unprotected sex is a sin in our society, methamphetamine abuse is a modern plague, and obesity threatens a generation. As an American researcher who specializes in behaviors supposedly related to acquiring AIDS told the *New York Times*, "There is risk going on out there." There isn't really a lot of AIDS going on out there, not in the United States. But we aren't meant to be concerned with AIDS. It's risk we are supposed to worry about.

Epidemic panics come and go, and now the hysteria can be independent of actual disease outbreaks. The current panic over crystal meth revisits the themes common to historical epidemics of "demon rum": the seductive elixir, the perilous insatiability of human appetites, the resulting intoxication—the drunkenness, in this view, is not just the effect of the dangerous broth but also a moral stupor that leads the user to consume more and more, until he succumbs. This was the story told of heroin, cocaine, pot, crack, and Ecstasy, before it was reprised for crystal meth. With meth, a new ingredient helps to identify the drug as demonic: it is allegedly related to HIV risk. If crystal meth invites risk, then it is not only bad because it is addictive and leads the unsuspecting down the path to ruin: it's bad because it is risky. Not that there is any evidence that meth users are actually more susceptible to acquiring the AIDS virus. But the facts are not relevant here. There's a lot of risk going on out there.

THE DISTANCING OF REAL DISEASE

Anxiety about modernity also blinds us to the truth of real suffering. The most serious of real epidemic diseases occur predominantly outside America and Europe nowadays—malaria, TB, sleeping sickness, diarrhea, even AIDS. These problems seem less and less relevant to us. We resort, suddenly, to the epidemiologist's definition of "epidemic," reminding ourselves that the toll those diseases take does not exceed expectation and therefore they are not epidemic but "endemic." Or we call them "global epidemics," which means, often, "not our problem."

When we talk about disease outbreaks today, the discussion is more often about what might happen and what we must be prepared for than about the massive mortality that is already happening, albeit not in our own part of the world. We are supposed to be prepared for a pandemic of avian flu, although it seems highly unlikely that there will ever be one. We are supposed to be prepared for a pandemic of some kind of influenza, because the flu watchers, the people who make a living studying the virus and who need to attract continued grant funding to keep studying it, must persuade the funding agencies of the urgency of fighting a coming plague. There is no particular reason to think that there will ever be another epidemic of flu to equal the 1918 outbreak, and no reason to think that if any flu strain does manage to go global it will be any worse than the garden-variety strains that come around every winter. But the forecasting of harm is essential to creating an epidemic story now, and it is indispensable for managing our fearful reactions. The prediction of a dire future always takes the form of a story that emphasizes our flaws: lack of preparedness, disorganization, or just disbelief. The augury on epidemics always demands that we take action to fix these flaws, as when New York's health commissioner talked about "complacency" to explain why he created a public panic about a nonexistent outbreak of AIDS in 2005 and when the State Department warned against complacency in combating the nonexistent bird flu epidemic in 2008. The epidemic story has to include the deep-down fault—complacency, susceptibility, blindness to risk—as well as the dangerous new product (crystal meth, vaccines, processed food, etc.), unbridled appetites, and a failure of vigilance.

The ratcheting up of fear by forecasting epidemics today contrasts with the pattern of the past, when preexisting fears were displaced onto epidemics. Politicians, preachers, and pundits made use of epidemics in that way. They justified people's underlying antipathy to foreigners, dark-skinned people, or sexual transgressors, renaming it as a reasonable response to the danger posed by real disease threats like plague, cholera, polio, or VD. They played on those latent fears to create programs that would help their political cause or their moral crusade. But in the plague era or the cholera years, it would have been irrational not to be afraid of the epidemic in the first place, given how deadly it was. The art of managing fear for political or moral ends involved redirecting existing fear, so that terror at the possibility of social collapse or genuine hatred toward Irish immigrants could masquerade as a normal reaction to a real epidemic. Today, the fear has to be ignited in the first place, and for that the epidemic has to be concocted. Real epidemics, like MRSA, don't seem to carry sufficient rhetorical power—they don't allow for enough manipulation of the public. It is more effective to create the obesity epidemic, the bioterrorist-borne smallpox outbreak, or the crystal-meth plague. The *possible* epidemic is rich in potential for managing the public.

Science should help clarify the distinction between outbreaks of real disease and imagined epidemics. But science is in no position to address the difference. At least in the United States, a scientist cannot live without grant money. To get grant money, a scientist has to produce new knowledge. And knowledge about an epidemic is only recognizable if it fits with the imagined version, if it tells the story of a disease of interest in a way that is recognizable. The story could be avian flu, AIDS, SARS, or a new disease, or it could be obesity, metabolic syndrome, bioterrorism, or even satanic ritual abuse. The key ingredient is that the story (it is called the "justification" or "rationale" in a researcher's proposal for grant funding) must generate enough fear of dangerous health consequences to persuade the funding agencies to open their pocketbooks. The researcher will not want to bet that she can obtain grant funding for studies to show that being overweight is usually benign or that most crystal-meth users suffer no long-lasting health problems from their habit. She won't get grants by seeking to show that avian flu is very unlikely to produce a human epidemic. She would be shooting herself in the foot. It would be far wiser for her to plan her investigations to demonstrate what the funders expect. Grant money is for generating knowledge only of a certain kind: facts that fit the story, that can be understood in terms of the epidemic as imagined.

NATURE'S BLOODY TEETH IN
THE MODERN WORLD

Nature remains more violent and deadly than any human contrivance, no matter how scary technology might seem. The more sophisticated human technology gets and the more complicated our society seems, the more anxious we become that technology will be our undoing. There is no reason to believe that people will suddenly stop feeling increasingly intense anxiety as technology gets more and more stunningly capable of altering nature. But nature has always outdone our worst fears. It will continue to offer horrific surprises, no matter how awful we think that man-made weapons have become.

In a sense, as far as naturally occurring outbreaks of illness go, Hippocrates had as good an explanation as any that has been advanced since. There is a mysterious coincidence of diseases with places. We can take a lot of the mystery out now, given the expansion of understanding that science has brought us. But we cannot remove all of the mystery. Hippocrates (and Napoleon) knew that geography is destiny. Where you are—"where" in its most complete sense, including whom you interact with and how—determines what sorts of diseases will be your lot. The nineteenth-century miasmatists were wrong about cholera, but they recognized some of the essentialness of place in the matter of disease outbreaks. Today, we might benefit from taking a page from the miasmatists' book. We might acknowledge that disease outbreaks are fundamentally unpredictable in detail—nature remains bloody in tooth and claw—and stop seeking out highly simplistic explanations. We might even recognize the most fundamental truth about disease outbreaks: they are worst for people who are worst off.

The current approach to global warming is an example of both what we could stop doing and what we might begin. We should stop listening to scientists who claim to be able to foresee the future. Many disease-control scientists are forecasting future calamity now, predicting catastrophic flu outbreaks or joining the bioterrorism-preparedness crusade. We should leave the job of seeing the future to the mystics, prophets, and fortune-tellers. On the other hand, we might demand that our scientists and officials look at disease outbreaks with as much nuance and attention to detail as the environmental scientists bring to the problem of global warming. Nobody seriously thinks that a single intervention is going to reverse the warming of the earth. And nobody claims that any one element—industrial pollution, the automobile, or rain forest destruction—is responsible. We understand the earth as a complex system, an ecosystem. Why not be as nuanced about illness?

What we think is likely to happen in nature almost never does. Avian flu remains a disease of birds. It has killed more than two hundred humans worldwide as of this writing, but it has not killed the millions of people that the pandemic scenarios predicted. The predictions that the prevalence of infection with the AIDS virus would rise to reach 50 percent everywhere (as it had among "fast-lane" gay men in San Francisco in the early '80s) never came true. The increase of tuberculosis cases in the early 1990s briefly stopped the long-term decline in TB mortality in the United States, leading to predictions that TB would roar back to be the dire health problem it had been before there were antibiotics. But TB's "resurgence" turned out to be a blip. Most of the great scares of recent years have not panned out. Flesh-eating bacteria, West Nile virus, SARS, bioterrorism—all turned out to be possible and some were even responsible for some deaths, but none has been the new plague.

Whatever disease causes the next great outbreak, we won't see it coming. The ones we do see are never as hard to handle as the epidemic that the watchers claim to see in our future. The ones that we will not be able to handle can't be foreseen. We concoct stories to make sense of our dread—but the real outbreaks are never really what we imagine the epidemic to be. This means that we are right to be fearful, but we are wrong if we think that any particular reading of risk or shift in our "risk behavior," any adjustment in our patterns of socializing, or any prohibition against air travel is going to stop the next great plague.

Nature terrifies us. Disfigurement horrifies us. Death we dread and disorder we fear. We cannot dispense with the terror, the horror, or the dread. When death rumbles around wantonly, we tell a story to make sense of it. And when no deadly disease is rampant, we create our own horror stories, scare ourselves beyond the simple fear of our own or our society's demise. We seem to need this story of risk—the story of invasion, suspect strangers, occult contamination, or hereditary susceptibilities. We can load outbreaks of contagion with the concerns of the day in order to tell ourselves this story, but when there is no outbreak we tell the story anyway. Most of us do not die in plagues. Most of the time, plagues do not happen. Yet without the story of the next plague, we would deny ourselves a main outlet for our dread. The key is to find ways to face our dread without being manipulated into doing what we do not need to do, buying what we do not need to buy, or fearing the people who represent no real threat.

There might or might not be another great plague, a rival to the Black Death, cholera, or the 1918 flu. People will likely talk about social problems through the story of a new epidemic. The concept of an epidemic as an outbreak of a recognizable disease had a seven-hundred-year run, going back to the plague outbreak of the fourteenth century. Now the epidemic is returning to its earlier, larger meaning: something that is intimately related to us as a people and to our home as a place. It has come to denote the crisis that tells us who we are, what's wrong with us, and what we think we need to fix.

The ancient Greek meaning of "epidemic"—native, homegrown—really applies to the concept of the epidemic itself: telling the story of spreading danger, errant habits, imminent social collapse, and so forth seems to be part of us, a native characteristic. The epidemic story is part of who we are.

—✺—

We can let the epidemic have its wandering and various meanings. But the epidemic is, in a way, always a story, a narrative, an account that is meant (by its teller) to take a stand about what she or he thinks is a problem, to propose, even if subtly, what should be done differently. We might remember this when we are told that we must accept more surveillance or buy new products in order to ward off epidemic threats. When we believe that tax dollars must be spent to fund biopreparedness exercises because foreign terrorists might create smallpox epidemics, that we should fear promiscuous homosexuals because they spread "superbugs," that we should not vaccinate our children lest they become autistic, or that we should be careful about befriending fat people because the obesity epidemic threatens our welfare, we might ask what it is we are afraid of. We might consider who benefits by forecasting the new threat, by configuring risk as a consequence of tolerating Islamic fundamentalists, men having sex with men, government immunization programs, or human appetite. We might wonder whether we gain anything more than momentary peace of mind by buying the epidemic story as it is being told. Most of all, we might consider whether there are ways to alleviate the suffering and forestall the premature death that really does occur in the world, rather than still our anxieties by blaming someone for exposing us to risk.

The epidemic story is filled, always, with the anxieties that make us tick. It's a story we should read conscientiously, aware of who is telling it and what the message is, bearing in mind that the risk-free life is a mirage.

ACKNOWLEDGMENTS

This book began as a conversation with my friend and colleague Ann Williams, about a course she taught at the Yale School of Nursing in the mid-1990s. The course was called "AIDS as Metaphor," and our conversation led to a series of discussions on the meanings attached to illness. I am indebted to Ann for that and many enlightening conversations over the years. Later, the directors of a Fordham University literary conference, "Malady in Literature," in April 2000 were generous enough to allow an epidemiologist to suggest that the scientific account of disease and the creative writer's account of disease fertilize each other in informative ways. Between those beginnings and the published book, many people have influenced my thinking and otherwise helped this project along.

Charles E. Rosenberg's essay "What Is an Epidemic: AIDS in Historical Perspective" first laid out the argument I make here about the epidemic as social narrative. The work of other historians in a similar vein influenced my thinking, notably that of Allan Brandt and Howard Markel.

Thoughtful discussions with many of my students at Hunter College enlightened my approach to aspects of the material. I am grateful to all the students of my "Imagined Epidemic" course and my courses on ethics in public health. I especially thank Ray Stridiron, Rachel Barbour, Sarah Donan Hirsch, Vera Hau, Katie Adamides, Nataliya Kukil, Michael Spiegelhalter, Liat Krawczyk, Patricia Winter, and

Ken Levin. Candice Belanoff did informative research on media coverage of toxic shock syndrome. Monica Serrano's extraordinary research on the panic involving the HIV "superbug" illuminated aspects of AIDS policy discussed in chapter 6. Stephanie Donald's insights regarding Magic Johnson and his women influenced my argument in Chapter 6.

I am indebted to many faculty colleagues at Hunter College. Elizabeth Beaujour encouraged me to develop courses based on my research and to offer them under the aegis of the Thomas Hunter Honors Program. Sandra Clarkson covered my administrative responsibilities to give me time to write. My colleagues in the Program on Urban Public Health offered insight into how people think about disease. I particularly thank Nick Freudenberg, Mark Goldberg, and David Kotelchuck for unfailing reminders about the social aspects of public health. Marilyn Auerbach consistently supported my scholarly research into the history of public health. Dean Laurie Sherwen and Provost Vita Rabinowitz generously released me from some teaching to allow time for research, and Hunter College provided travel funds so that I could visit libraries. Bernadette McCauley and Jack Levinson (the latter now at the College of the City of New York) were unstinting with their time for conversations. Tamara Green and Robert White helped with ancient Greek. Rebecca Connor gave me a valuable introduction to Gothic literature. Arlene Spark had many conversations with me on nutrition and obesity, and graciously reviewed manuscript material. Laura Cobus, head of the Health Professions Library at Hunter College, accommodated many requests for books and articles, and located even the hardest-to-find ones. Responsibility for misinterpretations or mistakes is mine alone, however.

Outside of Hunter College, Dr. Vic Sidel shared his thinking on bioterrorism, Helen Epstein engaged in many rich discussions on public health with me, especially on AIDS and Africa. Rachel Hadas encouraged me to pursue the connections between literary accounts and science. Lennard Davis has long been a conversation partner in wide-ranging discussions on the encounter of biology with culture. Ernest Drucker introduced me to a view of epidemiology in social and policy context that has remained fundamental to my research. Dr. Polly Thomas enlightened me as to how official agencies approached AIDS in the 1980s. Eileen Sullivan brought me the Airplane Man story. Ron and Marilyn Bush provided hospitality on several occasions while I worked in libraries in Oxford and London. TIAA-CREF supported an early lecture whose success led to much of the work presented here. Editors at *The American Scholar* (Anne Fadiman, William Whitworth, Robert Wilson) and *Virginia Quarterly Review* (Ted Genoways) helped me clarify my thinking on bioterrorism and AIDS, and published my essays on these topics. Randall Bytwerk kindly granted permission to reproduce a cartoon from *Der Stürmer*, in Chapter 5. Quotations from Camus's *The Plague* appear courtesy of Random House.

I am also grateful to librarians and archivists at the Bodleian Library at Oxford, the Houghton Library at Harvard, the rare books and manuscripts collection of Butler Library at Columbia University, the British Library manuscripts room, the New York Public Library, the Hunter College Main Library, and the archives of the Royal Society of Medicine in London.

I am most grateful to my agent, Lisa Bankoff, and her colleague Tina Wexler, who helped shape the idea for the book. Meredith Smith and the editing team at Perseus Books put the manuscript in shape. I am particularly indebted to Mark Sorkin for his painstaking reading of the manuscript and considerable help in making it clearer. This book would not have been what it is without the vision of Susan Weinberg or the clarity, effort, and patience of my editor at PublicAffairs, Morgen Van Vorst.

I thank Analena Alcabes and Sam and Aaron Ghitelman for their support. Above all, I thank Judith Baumel for ideas, colloquy, criticism, forbearance, encouragement, companionship, devotion, and probably much that I haven't yet appreciated.

NOTES

CHAPTER 1: THE SENSE OF AN EPIDEMIC

7   **And which of the gods:** Homer, *The Iliad*, trans. Samuel Butler (London: Longmans, Green, and Co., 1898), lines 10–15.

7   **the agency claims:** Eric Lichtblau and Nicholas Wade, "FBI Details Anthrax Case, but Doubts Remain," *New York Times*, August 19, 2008. A summary and timeline of the outbreak and investigation is available at http://topics.nytimes.com/top/reference/timestopics/subjects/a/anthrax/index.html (downloaded August 24, 2008).

7   **international convention:** U.S. State Department, "Convention on the Prohibition of the Development, Production and Stockpiling of Bacteriological (Biological) and Toxin Weapons and on Their Destruction," at http://www.state.gov/t/ac/trt/4718.htm (downloaded October 24, 2008); Mark Wheelis, Lajos Rozsa, and Malcolm Dando, eds., *Deadly Cultures: Biological Weapons Since 1945* (Cambridge: Harvard University Press, 2006), chaps. 1 and 2.

8   **five died:** "Developments in Anthrax Scare of 2001," Associated Press, September 27, 2003, reprinted at http://www.ph.ucla.edu/epi/bioter/developmentsanthrax.html (downloaded January 7, 2008).

8   **putting people in danger:** Elisa Harris, "The Killers in the Lab," *New York Times*, August 12, 2008, A21.

8   **arrived by letter:** Centers for Disease Control and Prevention, "Update: Investigation of Bioterrorism-Related Anthrax and Adverse Events from Antimicrobial Prophylaxis," *Morbidity and Mortality Weekly Report* 50, no. 44 (November 9, 2001): 973–976.

8   **symposium at Harvard's School of Public Health:** Alvin Powell, "SPH Bioterrorism Discussion Timely," *Harvard Gazette*, November 1, 2001.

9   **Pundits painted:** Hoover Institution film, *Nowhere to Run, Nowhere to Hide: Bioterrorism*, May 1998.

9   **in a domed stadium:** Walter Laqueur, *The New Terrorism: Fanaticism and the Arms of Mass Destruction* (New York: Oxford University Press, 1999), 64.

9   **Ditto malaria:** R. W. Snow, M. H. Craig, C. R. J. C. Newton, R. W. Stekete, "The Public Health Burden of Plasmodium Falciparum Malaria in Africa: Deriving the Number," working paper no. 11, Disease Control Priorities Project at the Fogarty International Center, National Institutes of Health, August 2003, cited in Joel G. Breman, Anne Mills, Robert W. Snow, Jo-Ann Mulligan, Christian Lengeler, Kamini Mendis, Brian Sharp, Chantal Morel, Paola Marchesini, Nicholas J. White, Richard W. Steketee, and Ogobara K. Doumbo, "Conquering Malaria," *Disease Control Priorities in Developing Countries*, 2nd ed. (New York: Oxford University Press, 2006), 413–432. At http://www.dcp2.org/pubs/DCP/21/ (downloaded November 29, 2008).

10   **Hippocrates drew:** Hippocrates, *On Airs, Waters, and Places*, trans. Francis Adams. This text is available from Internet Classics Archive at http://classics.mit.edu/Hippocrates/airwatpl.3.3.html (downloaded January 11, 2009). I have provided modern spellings of medical terms.

11   *epidemiou* **in ancient times:** According to the Liddell-Scott-Jones Lexicon, available at www.perseus.tufts.edu.

11   **Homer refers:** Paul M. V. Martin and Estelle Martin-Granel, "2,500-year Evolution of the Term Epidemic," *Emerging Infectious Diseases*, June 2006, http://www.cdc.gov/ncidod/EID/vol12no06/05-1263.htm.

12   **other recognizable conditions:** See, for instance, George Rosen, *A History of Public Health*, expanded ed. (Baltimore: Johns Hopkins University Press, 1993), chap. 1.

13   **tried to make sense:** This argument is advanced by Charles-Edward Amory Winslow, *The Conquest of Epidemic Disease: A Chapter in the History of Ideas*, paperback ed. (Madison: University of Wisconsin, 1980), 54; following F. H. Garrison, *An Introduction to the History of Medicine*, 4th ed. (Philadelphia: Saunders, 1929).

13   **a moral meaning:** Martin and Martin-Granel, "2,500-year Evolution."

13   **destruction of human life:** Thucydides, *Histories*, trans. P. J. Rhodes, book 2, sect. 47; modified by G. E. R. Lloyd, *In the Grip of Disease: Studies in the Greek Imagination* (New York: Oxford University Press, 2003), 137. I have translated *nosos* here as "disease" in lieu of Lloyd's "plague," to capture a distinction between malady per se and malady delivered en masse.

13   **The plague is said to have come:** Ibid.

14   **Virgil invokes:** Virgil, *Eclogues-Georgics-Aeneid 1–6*, trans. H. Rushton Fairclough, revised by G. P. Gould (Cambridge: Harvard University Press, 1999), *Georgics* book 3, lines 471–472.

14   **the adder:** Ibid., line 419.

14   **cataclysmic outbreak:** In fact, the French derivative of *plagare* is *plaie*, meaning merely a wound or sore; the German derivative, *Plage*, means only a nuisance.

15   **the work of demons:** Francesco Bottin, Giovanni Santinello, Philip Weller, and C. W. T. Blackwell, eds., *Models of the History of Philosophy* (Boston: Kluwer Academic Publishers, 1993), 185. Also Joseph Jastrow, *Wish and Wisdom* (New York: Appleton-Century, 1935), and Lucien Levy-Bruhl, *Primitives and the Supernatural* (London: Allen and Unwin, 1936); both cited in Winslow, *Conquest of Epidemic Disease*, 1980 ed., chap. 1.

15   **judgments about disease:** See Winslow, especially chaps. 1 and 2.

15   **the flesh that touches:** Nosson Scherman, ed., *The Tanach, Stone Edition*, 2nd ed. (New York: Mesorah, 1998).

16   **I will send a pestilence:** This translation from Scherman, *Tanach* (New York: Mesorah, 1996), 311.

16   **David . . . chooses:** *Tanakh: The Holy Scriptures*, trans. Jewish Publication Society (Philadelphia: JPS, 1985), 513.

18   **flluxe or other ipedemye:** *Oxford English Dictionary*, 240. The citation is from the *Paston Letters*, 703 III 59.

CHAPTER 2: PLAGUE

21   **There have been as many plagues as wars:** Albert Camus, *The Plague*, trans. Stuart Gilbert, 1948 (New York: Vintage, 1991), 37.

21   **apocalyptic scenarios:** James Kinsella, *Covering the Plague: AIDS and the American Media* (New Brunswick: Rutgers University Press, 1989), 54; Dennis Altman, *AIDS in the Mind of America* (Garden City: Anchor, 1986), 17–19. Kinsella cites a September 1982 syndicated article by United Press International reporter Jan Ziegler; Altman names other 1982 news articles and gives August 9, 1982, as the date of the first article about "gay plague"; a *Newsweek* story in August 1982 was titled "Homosexual Plague Strikes New Victims."

23   ***Yersinia pestis:*** James Chin, ed., *Control of Communicable Diseases Manual*, 17th ed. (Washington, DC: American Public Health Association, 1999).

23   **in medieval Europe:** The evidence for continuous rat-flea involvement even in the largest plague outbreak of all time, and even when plague was spreading most rapidly, is summarized in Ole J. Bendictow, *The Black Death 1346–1353: The Complete History* (Rochester: Boydell Press, 2004), 11–34.

24   **a million homes:** Laurie Garrett, *Betrayal of Trust: The Collapse of Global Public Health* (New York: Hyperion, 2000), 19.

24   **several hundred cases:** Indian Ministry of Health data released October 10, 1994, reported in Garrett, *Betrayal of Trust*, 591.

24   **Subsequent salients:** Jacqueline Brossollet and Henri Mollaret, *Pourquoi la Peste? Le Rat, La Puce et Le Bubon* (Paris: Gallimard, 1994), 16–20; William H. McNeill, *Plagues and Peoples* (New York: Anchor, 1977), 109–116.

25   **passing through Constantinople:** For discussions of the arrival of plague, see Barbara Tuchman, *A Distant Mirror: The Calamitous 14th Century* (New York: Knopf, 1978), 92–94; Sheldon Watts, *Epidemics and History: Disease, Power, and Imperialism* (New Haven: Yale University Press, 1997), 8–10; and Brossollet and Mollaret, *Pourquoi la Peste?* 32–33; McNeill devotes much of his fourth chapter to an exploration of the arrival of plague as a manifestation of the Mongol Empire's influence, *Plagues and Peoples*, 132–150.

25   **few plague-sick travelers:** Chin, *Control of Communicable Diseases*.

25   **began in China:** Robert Gottfried, *The Black Death: Natural and Human Disaster in Medieval Europe* (New York: Free Press, 1983), 35.

25   **origin in central Asia:** McNeill *Plagues and Peoples*; Benedictow, *The Black Death*.

26   **usual countryside cycle:** Jean-Noel Biraben, "Current Medical and Epidemiological Views on Plague," in Paul Slack, ed., *The Plague Reconsidered: A New Look at Its Origins and Effects in 16th and 17th Century England* (Matlock, UK: Social Population Studies, 1977), 25–36; Norman Gratz, "Rodent Reservoirs & Flea Vectors of Natural Foci of Plague," in *Plague Manual: Epidemiology, Distribution, Surveillance and Control* (World Health Organization, 1999), 65–67, text available at http://www.who.int/csr/resources/publications/plague/WHO_CDS_CSR_EDC_99_2_EN/en/ (downloaded January 11, 2009).

26   **wild mammals:** This theory was put forth by McNeill, *Plagues and Peoples*, 111. It is sound, for three reasons. First, the black rat is an epizootic host for plague bacilli, not an enzootic one: plague kills rats; the rat population, while it could move *Y. pestis* as it migrated during rat epizootics, would not have sustained *Y. pestis* infection at high prevalence for very long. It is well known that plague is enzootic among wild rodents in central Asia (for example, see Jacques Ruffié and Jean-Charles Sournia, *Les Épidémies dans l'Histoire de l'Homme* [Paris: Flammarion, 1984], 11; the earliest field biology research on the topic of which I am aware was reported in N. P. Mironov, "The Past Existence of Foci of Plague in the Steppes of Southern Europe," *Journal of Hy-*

giene, Epidemiology, Microbiology and Immunology 29 (1958): 1193–
1198. Second, it concurs with our knowledge that other pathogens
cross species barriers through various forms of intermixing among animal species, including sexual contact, sharing living space, and eating
one another (see, for instance, Stephen L. Morse, *Emerging Viruses*
[New York: Oxford University Press, 1996]; Madeline Drexler, *The
Menace of Emerging Infections* [New York: Penguin, 2003]). Third, it is
consistent with historians' suggestion that plague is ancient in India
and moved out of the subcontinent and into the steppes of northern
central Asia only just before it entered Europe (see, for instance, Mc-
Neill, *Plagues and Peoples*, 111–112 and chap. 4).

26   **it could spread widely:** Bendictow, *The Black Death*, chap. 1.

27   **This is an example:** Quoted in Watts, *Epidemics and History*, 1.

27   **In Ireland:** Tuchman, *A Distant Mirror*, 95–105; quoting from Philip
Ziegler, *The Black Death* (New York: Harper and Row, 1969). Tuchman's account contains numerous references to fourteenth-century beliefs that the epidemic represented divine disfavor.

27   **a matter of disagreement:** Charles-Edward Amory Winslow, *The Conquest of Epidemic Disease: A Chapter in the History of Ideas*, paperback
ed. (Madison: University of Wisconsin Press, 1980), 99 ff.

28   **spiritual failing:** A. Lynn Martin, *Plague? Jesuit Accounts of Epidemic
Disease in the 16th Century* (Kirksville, MO: Truman State University
Press, 1996), 98. Martin points out that the Protestant view discrimi-
nated physical health from spiritual well-being, holding that post-
Reformation Christians were therefore less able to embrace human
agency as a cure for spiritually inspired illness.

28   **an expression of divine punishment:** Susan Sontag, *Illness as Metaphor
and AIDS and its Metaphors* (Anchor/Doubleday, 1990), 43.

29   **undermine Christian society:** This argument is based on the studies of
Carlo Ginzburg. See *Ecstasies: Deciphering the Witches' Sabbath*, trans.
Raymond Rosenthal (New York: Penguin, 1991).

29   **spiritual taint:** See Watts, *Epidemics and History*, chap. 2, 40–83; also
Ruffié and Sournia, *Les Épidémies*, 151–164, on the meanings of leprosy
to medieval Christians. Watts's extensive inquiry into the meaning of
leprosy in the Middle Ages and its relation to both the construction of
Western society and European empire building is insightful. He makes
the connection between the treatment of lepers and the treatment of
Jews.

29   **the leper "shall dwell apart":** Translation from the Rabbinical Assem-
bly, *Etz Hayim: Torah and Commentary* (New York: Jewish Publication
Society, 2001).

29   misidentified the disease: Watts, *Epidemics and History*, 40–48.

29   spiritual reform: This translation, and the interpretation, come from Nosson Scherman, ed., *The Tanach, Stone Edition*, 2nd ed. (New York: Mesorah, 1998), 272 ff.

30   behavior that signaled trouble: Watts, *Epidemics and History*, 49.

30   wear identifying insignia: J. N. Hays, *The Burdens of Disease: Epidemics and Human Response in Western History* (New Brunswick: Rutgers University Press, 2000), 20–29.

30   giving succor to the leper: Ibid.

31   avoid inadvertent contamination: Tuchman, *A Distant Mirror*, 112; Watts *Epidemics and History*, 55.

31   bedeviled: Joshua Trachtenberg, *The Devil and the Jews: The Medieval Conception of the Jew and its Relation to Modern Antisemitism* (Philadelphia: Jewish Publication Society, 1983), 20 ff.

31   envy, scorn, and resentment: Mordechai Breuer and Michael. Graetz, *Tradition and Enlightenment, 1600–1780* (New York: Columbia University Press, 1996), 13, cited in John Kelly, *The Great Mortality: An Intimate History of the Black Death, the Most Devastating Plague of All Time* (New York: HarperCollins, 2005), 236.

31   slaughtered every Jew: Tuchman, *A Distant Mirror*, 41.

32   a great number of lepers: Author's translation of Gillaume de Nangis, *Chroniques Capétiennes*, trans. from Latin by Francois Guizot (Clermont-Ferrand, France: Paleo, 2002), 2:181 ff.

32   Care of the Jews: Ibid.

32   not unusual in that era: J. Shatzmiller, "Les juifs de Provence pendant la Peste noire," *Revue des Etudes Juives* 133 (1974): 457–480, cited in John Kelly, *The Great Mortality*, 138.

33   posted in the cemetery: Tuchman gives the number of Jews murdered in Strasbourg as 2,000; Watts says 900.

33   burned to death: Brossollet and Mollaret, *Pourquoi la Peste?* 37.

33   mobs could attack Jews with impunity: Trachtenberg, *The Devil and the Jews*, 105.

33   Duke of Meissen instructed: The duke's order is described in the *Chronicum Parvum Dresdense*, cited in Norman Davies, *Europe: A History* (New York: Oxford University Press, 1996), 414.

34   "Rabbi Jacob" of Spain: Rosemary Horrox, *The Black Death* (Manchester: Manchester University Press, 1994).

34   poisons that Jews supposedly used: The account here of attacks on Jews in 1349 comes from Tuchman, *A Distant Mirror*, 113 ff.; Brossollet and Mollaret, *Pourquoi la Peste?* 36–37; and Trachtenberg, *The Devil and the*

Jews, 102–107. The killing of Jews was clearly not a civil war between followers of the church and proponents of a perceived heresy. The church was unbending in its suppression of the flagellant movement, an anarchist sect of believers who flogged themselves in public processionals, seeking to extirpate sin and purify their moral beings by scourging their own flesh. When the dualism of the Cathars (sometimes called the Albigensian heresy) had threatened the church's authority in the early 1200s, King Philip Augustus of France, along with allies like Simon de Montfort, suppressed them violently. Similarly, the pope excommunicated the Waldensian pauper-preachers in 1184, and the Fourth Lateran Council of 1215 anathemized them. See Stephen O'Shea, *The Perfect Heresy: The Revolutionary Life and Death of the Medieval Cathars* (New York: Walker and Co., 2001). Also Ronald F. Malan, "Waldensian History: A Brief Sketch," April 2004, http://homepages.rootsweb.com/ ~waldense/history.htm#19 (downloaded June 26, 2007).

34   **not fully systematized:** John Cartwright, "Poems of Science: Chaucer's Doctor of Physick," *Education Forum* 46, February 2004.

35   **burning herbs:** Tuchman, *A Distant Mirror*, 106–107.

35   **Chaucer, writing at the time:** Geoffrey Chaucer, *The Canterbury Tales*, General Prologue, lines 425–428, in *The Works of Geoffrey Chaucer*, 2nd ed., F. N. Robinson, ed. (Boston: Houghton Mifflin, 1957), 21.

35   **Some historians believe:** The historian Jeremy Cohen points out that piety would have been untenable for middle-class Christians by the middle of the 1400s had it only been approachable by retreating from worldly life; cloistered monasticism had worked to demonstrate piety to a feudal world, but it could not be the only option available for the devout in a much more commercial era. The church, for its part, couldn't afford to demand that its constituents hew closely to the old fashion, since by the thirteenth century it risked losing their allegiance to new heresies. The church modernized piety, creating two new orders of friars: the Dominicans and the Franciscans. These orders, more engaged with the world than the older Benedictines and Cistercians, drew from the middle class and were middle class in their predispositions. For a full examination of movements within the late medieval church and their ramifications with respect to nonbelievers, see Jeremy Cohen, *The Friars and the Jews: The Evolution of Medieval Anti-Judaism* (Ithaca: Cornell University Press, 1982), 34–44.

36   **Jews were expelled . . . in 1424:** Trachtenberg, *The Devil and the Jews*, 107.

36   **in 1488 . . . converted Jew:** Ibid.

36   **plague and penitence:** The connection between plague and penitence was ancient. Christine M. Boeckl notes that in the fourth century, Eusebius, bishop of Caesarea in the Middle East, professed that to die of pestilence is to die a martyr. See Boeckl, *Images of Plague and Pestilence: Iconology and Iconography* (Kirksville, MO: Truman State University Press, 2000), 41.

36   **Gregory of Tours:** Author's translation, from Brossollet and Mollaret, *Pourquoi la Peste?*, p. 26.

37   **The Jesuits knew . . . divine sacrament:** Martin, *Plague?* 95–98.

37   **displaying of holy relics:** Ibid., 101.

37   **"I murdered some of them":** Gerard Robinson, "Kramer Aims at HIV, Tina," *New York Blade* online, November 12, 2004, http://www.nyblade .com/2004/11-12/news/national/kramer.cfm (downloaded August 2, 2007).

38   **vain attempts of pitiable infants:** Johannes Nohl, *The Black Death: A Chronicle of the Plague Compiled from Contemporary Sources*, trans. C. H. Clarke (London: Unwin, 1961), 21.

38   **Faith, we are meant to understand:** Boeckl, *Images of Plague and Pestilence*, 26.

38   **Gargiulo was a health deputy:** Bernardo de Dominici, *Vite dei pittori, scultori ed architetti napoletane*, vol. 3 (Naples: Tipografia Trani, 1840).

39   **The work was commissioned:** Horst Ziermann, *Matthias Grünewald* (New York: Prestel Verlag, 2001), 78.

39   **how physical illness was understood:** Georg Scheja, *The Isenheim Altarpiece*, trans. Robert Erich Wolf (New York: Harry N. Abrams, 1969).

39   **swelling of the skin or desquamation:** Ziermann, *Matthias Grünewald.*

39   **the poorest of the poor:** Ibid., 78.

40   **brick-red cloth of martyrdom:** Ibid., 103–104.

40   **could be read in Jesus' life:** Scheja, *The Isenheim Altarpiece*, 66.

40   **thin and easily crossed:** Hilde Schmölzer, *Die Pest in Wien* (Berlin: Verlag der Nation, 1988), 140.

40   **recipes that might be:** Royal College of Physicians, *Certain Necessary Directions as well for the Cure of the Plague as for Preventing the Infection, with Many Easie Medicines of Small Charge* (London: John Bill and Christopher Barker, 1665).

40   **remedies offered for use:** James L. Matterer, "17th Century English Recipes," http://www.godecookery.com/engrec/engrec.html#top (downloaded November 29, 2007). These recipes are transcribed from primary sources.

41   **clean the streets:** Francis Herring, *Certaine Rules, Directions, or Advertisements for This Time of Pestilentiall Contagion* (London: William Jones, 1625, reprinted New York: Da Capo, 1973).

41 **banned trade with Tortosa:** Miquel Parets, *A Journal of the Plague Year: The Diary of the Barcelona Tanner Miquel Parets* 1651, trans. James S. Amelang (New York: Oxford University Press, 1991).

41 **a real public, in the sense:** This argument is based on that of Jürgen Habermas, *The Structural Transformation of the Public Sphere*, trans. Thomas Berger (Cambridge: MIT Press, 1998), chap. 1. However, Habermas ignores the role of plague itself in developing what he calls the "public sphere."

42 **the city proper:** Gottfried, *The Black Death*, 48; Rosen, *A History of Public Health* (Baltimore: Johns Hopkins University Press, 1993), 43.

42 **forty days:** The modern word "quarantine" comes from the Italian *quarantina giorni*, designating this forty-day period. But even in the late 1700s, the period of sequestration at some spots varied with the point of origin and degree of suspicion about incoming shipping. According to historian Hilde Schmölzer (*Die Pest in Wien*, 1985), in 1770 the Austro-Hungarian Empire required twenty-one days for people entering from the east with bills of good health and forty-two days for those coming from plague-infested territories, and it seems that similar selectivity was in use at the Marseilles plague station as late as 1797. Joel Barlow claimed in a letter to the U.S. secretary of state in August 1797 that ships that had experienced a plague outbreak on board were quarantined for sixty to ninety days, whereas those with a clean bill of health but which had put in at a "Mahometan" port stayed for eighteen to twenty-five days, the exact period up to the discretion of the commissioner of health of the port. Barlow was an unreliable reporter, but he had commercial reasons to make this claim, and it seems likely to have been true. Barlow Letters, series I, vol. 4, Houghton Library, Harvard.

42 **banned from Pistoia:** *Gli Ordinamenti Sanitari del Comune di Pistoia contro la Pestilenza del 1348*, translated and excerpted by Horrox, *The Black Death*, 194 ff.

43 **for westward transport:** Schmölzer, *Die Pest in Wien*, 153–157.

43 **expelled from Milanese lands:** Horrox, *The Black Death*.

43 **houses stricken by plague be walled up:** Carlo Cipolla, "Per la Storia delle Epidemie in Italia," *Rivista Storica Italiana* 75 (1963), cited in Gottfried, *The Black Death*, 49.

43 **permitting troops to shoot individuals:** Biraben, *Les Hommes et la Peste en France et dans les Pays Européens et Méditerraneéns* (Paris: Mouton, 1976), cited by Watts, *Epidemics and History*, 23.

43 **twenty-one plague ordinances:** Stephen Porter, *The Great Plague* (Stroud, UK: Phoenix Mill, 1999), 16.

43   city of Rouen appointed men: Brossollet and Mollaret, *Pourquoi la Peste?* 39.

44   official edicts: Porter, *The Great Plague*, 14.

44   red cross painted by the door: Brossollet and Mollaret, *Pourquoi la Peste?* 40.

44   carry a white stick whenever they left the house: Paul Slack, *The Impact of Plague in Tudor and Stuart England* (Boston: Routledge and Kegan Paul, 1985), 201.

44   official watchmen to use force: Porter, *The Great Plague*, 16.

44   Plague taxes: R. S. Duplessis, *Lille and the Dutch Revolt: Urban Stability in an Era of Revolution 1500–1582* (Cambridge: Cambridge University Press, 1991) and J. H. Thomas, *Town Government in the Sixteenth Century* (New York: Kelley, 1969), both cited in Porter, *The Great Plague*, 13–14.

44   taxed during any time of plague: Slack, *The Impact of Plague*, 209–211.

45   buried as fast as they accumulated: Jean de Venette, quoted in Gottfried, *The Black Death*, 56.

45   too many deaths for the church bells to be tolled: Cited in Tuchman, *A Distant Mirror*, 95, 97.

45   no one knew where to turn: Ibid., 99–100.

45   no priest could be found to take confession: Quoted in William Naphy and Andrew Spicer, *The Black Death: A History of Plagues 1345–1730* (Charleston, SC: Tempus, 2000), 39.

45   first official compilation of death counts: Ibid., 34. Estimates of the mortality can be found in Susan Scott and Christopher J. Duncan, *Biology of Plagues: Evidence from Historical Populations* (Cambridge: Cambridge University Press, 2001).

45   other Italian localities began keeping similar bills: Ibid., 85.

45   London bills of mortality: Porter, *The Great Plague*, 15.

45   women called "searchers": John Graunt, *Reflections on the Weekly Bills of Mortality for the Cities of London and Westminster, and the Places Adjacent*, 1662 (edition printed for Samuel Speed, Fleet Street, 1665).

46   "rising of the lights": Ibid.

47   generally sparing men of means: Simon de Covino and John of Fordham, cited in Tuchman, *A Distant Mirror*, 98.

47   Venice lazaretto: *Informazioni sulle Isole Lazaretto Vecchio*, at http://194.243.104.176/websitimg_laguna/info/info_isola.asp?id=27 (downloaded August 29, 2008).

47   accommodation for the poor: Vincenzo Cavengo, *Il Lazzaretto: Storia di un Quartiere di Milano* (Milan: Nuove Edizioni Duomo, 1989), 54.

48   meant to be used for plague victims: Ibid., 48.

48   said to have accommodated 16,000 persons: Porter, *The Great Plague*, 10.

48   devil-combating immolations: Carlo Ginzburg, *Ecstasies: Deciphering the Witches' Sabbath*, trans. Raymond Rosenthal (New York: Penguin, 1991).

48   two men were hanged: Brossollet and Mollaret, *Pourquoi la Peste?* 37.

49   the Baltic region's: Johannes Nohl, *The Black Death: A Chronicle of the Plague Compiled from Contemporary Sources* (London: Unwin, 1961).

49   Vienna's: Schmölzer, *Die Pest in Wien*, 178; Nohl, *The Black Death*, 55.

50   eruptions in Astrakhan: John T. Alexander, *Bubonic Plague in Early Modern Russia: Public Health and Urban Disaster* (New York: Oxford University Press, 2003), 304.

50   better housing was so gradual: Porter, *The Great Plague*, 171.

50   helped limit the movements of infected fleas: The argument is made by the historian Paul Slack in "The Disappearance of Plague: An Alternative View," *Economic History Review* 34 (1981): 469–476.

50   *Pestkordon* at the Austro-Hungarian border: Schmölzer, *Die Pest in Wien*.

50   the black rat was replaced in Europe by the brown: Andrew A. Appleby, "The Disappearance of Plague: A Continuing Puzzle," *The Economic History Review* 33 (1980): 161–173.

51   the term *Black Death* was finally coined: Jean-Pierre Papon, *De la Peste, ou Époques Mémorables de ce Fléau* (Paris: Lavillette, 1800), cited in Brossollet and Mollaret, *Pourquoi la Peste?* 133. The English origin is given in the *Oxford English Dictionary*, 656. For German, Justus Friedrich Carl Hecker, *Der schwarze Tod im vierzehnten Jahrhundert: Nach den Quellen für Aerzte und gebildete Nichtärzte* (Berlin: Herbig, 1832).

52   which together kill almost as many Americans: Hsiang-Ching Kung, Donna L. Hoyert, Jiaquan Xu, and Sherry L. Murphy, "Deaths: Final Data for 2005," *National Vital Statistics Reports* 56 (2008): 5, table B.

52   jalapeño peppers: Nikhil Swaminathan, "Found: FDA Officials Link Salmonella Outbreak to Mexican-Grown Jalapeño," *Scientific American* online, July 22, 2008, at http://www.sciam.com/blog/60-second-science/post.cfm?id=found-fda-officials-link-salmonella-2008-07-22 (downloaded January 11, 2009).

CHAPTER 3: CHOLERA, POVERTY, AND THE POLITICIZED EPIDEMIC

53   Hippocrates, *On Winds*: Quoted in Wade Wright Oliver, *Stalkers of Pestilence: The Story of Man's Ideas of Infection* (Manchester, NH: Ayer Publishers, 1970), 28.

53   fevers of malaria were described: F. E. G. Cox, "History of Human Parasitology," *Clinical Microbiology Reviews* (October 2002): 595–612.

53   **Ground Zero:** R. M. Brackbill, L. E. Thorpe, L. DiGrande et al., "Surveillance for World Trade Center Disaster Health Effects Among Survivors of Collapsed and Damaged Buildings," *Morbidity and Mortality Weekly Report Surveillance Summary* 55, no. SS02 (April 7, 2006): 1–18; M. A. Perrin, L. DiGrande, K. Wheeler et al., "Differences in PTSD Prevalence and Associated Risk Factors Among World Trade Center Rescue and Recovery Workers," *American Journal of Psychiatry* 164 (2007): 1385–1394; Fire Department, City of New York, "World Trade Center Impacts on FDNY Rescue Workers: A Six-Year Assessment September 2001–September 2007," at http://www.nyc.gov/html/om/pdf/2007/wtc_health_impacts_on_fdny_rescue_workers_sept_2007.pdf (downloaded September 28, 2007).

53   **coal-dust-fouled air:** E. T. Wilkins, "Air Pollution Aspects of the London Fog of December 1952," *Quarterly Journal of the Royal Meteorological Society* 80, no. 344 (2006): 267–271.

54   **called a press conference:** Mike Stobbe, "Rare Tuberculosis Case Prompts Warning," Associated Press, May 29, 2007; Lauran Neergaard and Devlin Barrett, "U.S. Probes How TB Traveler Crossed Border," Associated Press, May 30, 2007; Lawrence Altman and John Schwartz, "Near Misses Allowed Man With Tuberculosis to Fly to and From Europe, Health Officials Say," *New York Times*, May 31, 2007. Additional reporting in *New York Times* articles by John Schwartz, June 2, 2007, and Lawrence Altman, July 5, 2007.

54   **his own convenience:** Editorial, "Isolating an Evasive TB Patient," *New York Times*, May 31, 2007.

54   **bloggers called him "selfish":** Shamalama, "How to Define Selfish," Common Folk Using Common Sense blog, at http://www.commonfolkusingcommonsense.com/2007/06/01/how-to-define-selfish/ (downloaded January 11, 2009).

54   **"undermining":** Michelle Malkin, "If We Can't Counter TB, How Can We Counter Terrorism?" at http://michellemalkin.com/2007/09/09/if-we-cant-counter-tb-how-can-we-counter-terrorism/ (downloaded January 11, 2009).

54   **filed suit against him:** Sean Farrell, "Nine File Suit Against TB-Infected Man," Associated Press, July 12, 2007.

55   **new Do Not Board program went into practice:** Amanda Gardner, "U.S. Barred 33 TB-infected People From Flying Over Past Year," *U.S. News and World Report*, HealthDay online, September 18, 2008, at http://health.usnews.com/articles/health/healthday/2008/09/18/us-barred-33-tb-infected-people-from-flying-over.html (downloaded October 30, 2008).

55   **fewer than 700:** TB mortality data from U.S. Centers for Disease
       Control and Prevention, "Reported Tuberculosis in the United States,
       2005," at http://www.cdc.gov/tb/surv/surv2005/default.htm (down-
       loaded September 17, 2007); total mortality data from U.S. National
       Center for Health Statistics, at http://www.cdc.gov/nchs/products/
       pubs/pubd/hestats/prelimdeaths05/prelimdeaths05.htm (downloaded
       September 18, 2007).

55   **only 815 in France, 849 in the U.K., and 595 in Germany:** World
       Health Organization, Global Tuberculosis Database, at http://www
       .who.int/globalatlas/dataQuery/default.asp (downloaded September
       17, 2007).

57   **Cholera occurs when:** Info on cholera from Abram S. Benenson, ed.,
       Control of Communicable Diseases in Man, 15th ed. (Washington, DC:
       American Public Health Association, 1990).

58   **cholera is treatable:** David A. Sack, R. Bradley Sack, G. Balakrish Nair,
       and A. K. Siddique, "Cholera," *Lancet* 363, no. 9404 (2004): 223–233.

58   **probably circulated continuously:** Charles E. Rosenberg, *The Cholera
       Years* (Chicago: University of Chicago Press, 1962), 1; William H.
       McNeill, *Plagues and Peoples* (New York: Anchor/Doubleday, 1977),
       230–232.

58   **subcontinent was heavily forested:** C. A. Bayley, *Indian Society and the
       Making of the British Empire*, cited in Sheldon Watts, *Epidemics and His-
       tory: Disease, Power, and Imperialism* (New Haven: Yale University
       Press, 1997), 181.

59   **encouraged to travel:** Watts, *Epidemics and History*, 179.

59   **10 million Bengalis:** Information on the fall of the Mughals comes
       from Watts, *Epidemics and History*, 176–182.

59   **first subcontinent-wide outbreak:** Ibid., 178.

59   **camel's hump:** Ibid., 171.

59   **eastward to China:** Ibid., 170–171.

59   **After cholera was carried to Muscat:** McNeil, *Plagues and Peoples*, 232.

59   **Russian troops returning:** Ibid., 232–233.

60   **Hungary lost 100,000 people:** Peter Baldwin, *Contagion and the State
       in Europe, 1830–1930* (Cambridge: Cambridge University Press, 1999),
       70–71.

60   **Hamburg and the other Hanseatic ports:** Geoffrey Marks and
       William K. Beatty, *Epidemic* (New York: Scribner, 1976).

60   **one-eighth of the population:** McNeil, *Plagues and Peoples*, 231.

60   **dozens of New Yorkers:** Rosenberg, *The Cholera Years*, 57.

60   **the northeastern coast:** Watts, *Epidemics and History*, 192–193.

60   **more than 31,000:** Ibid., 195.

60   **"Improvident habits are the ruin":** Herbert A. Smith, *A Letter to the Labouring Classes in Their Own Behalf* (London: W. Tyler, 1837), 5.

61   **Leeds more than doubled:** George Rosen, *A History of Public Health*, expanded ed. (Baltimore: Johns Hopkins University Press, 1993), 178.

61   **just six cities:** Dorothy Porter, *Health, Civilization and the State: A History of Public Health from Ancient to Modern Times* (New York: Routledge, 1999), 113.

61   **roughly 70 percent:** Rosen, *A History of Public Health*, 182.

61   **which included children:** Friedrich Engels, *The Condition of the Working Class in England* (New York: Oxford University Press, 1993), 160. Engels is citing a report by the Factory Inquiries Commission of 1833.

61   **Sanitation was sorely lacking:** Ibid., chap. 2, 36–76.

61   **emptied into the street:** Rosen, *A History of Public Health*, 181.

61   **Dickens describes:** Charles Dickens, *Hard Times* (Boston: Colonial Press, 1868); first American ed. (1854), 19.

61   **Berry Street:** Elizabeth Gaskell, *Mary Barton* (London: Oxford University Press, 1906), 66.

62   **poverty became threatening:** Porter, *Health, Civilization and the State*, 114–115.

62   **became highly mobile:** Ibid., 87–96. Porter explicates the political milieu creating this "mobile proletariat" and its effects.

62   **The Condition of the Working Class in England:** F. Engels, *The Condition of the Working Class in England* (New York: Oxford, 1993), 78.

63   **Marx and Engels wrote:** Karl Marx and Friedrich Engels, *The Communist Manifesto* (1848), trans. Samuel Moore (New York: Penguin, 2002), 223.

64   **the first workhouse:** Rosen, *A History of Public Health*, 171.

64   **7 million pounds:** Ibid., 172.

64   **the broadest aim:** Ibid., 176–177.

64   **gruel-and-water diet:** John Bowen, *A Refutation of Some of the Charges Against the Poor* (London: John Hatchard, 1837), 15.

65   **galvanized the British parliament:** Rosen, *A History of Public Health*, 192–196.

65   **about 2.5 million:** Kings College London, Center for Computing in the Humanities, table of historical population figures for London, at http://www.cch.kcl.ac.uk/legacy/teaching/av1000/numerical/problems/london/london-pop-table.html (downloaded February 23, 2008).

65   **More than three hundred:** John Paris and committee members, *Report of the Medical Council in Relation to the Cholera-Epidemic of 1854* (London: George E. Eyre & Wm. Spottiswoode, 1855).

65   **examples of epidemiologic investigation:** Snow recounts this and other research in his *On the Mode of Communication of Cholera*, avail-

able online at Dr. Ralph Frerichs's extensive Web collection on Snow. See http://www.ph.ucla.edu/epi/snow.html.

66   **the Nuisances Act:** It was based on the findings of the Medical Council of the General Board of Health; see "Chairman's Introduction," *Report of the Medical Council in Relation to the Cholera-Epidemic.*

66   **actually have helped spread cholera:** Steven Johnson, *The Ghost Map: The Story of London's Most Terrifying Epidemic and How It Changed Science, Cities, and the Modern World* (New York: Penguin, 2007), 117–121.

67   **"There are and can be":** Francis Bacon, *Novum Organum* (1620), section XIX, in James Spedding, Robert Leslie Ellis, Douglas Denon Heath, and William Rawley, *The Works of Frances Bacon* 4 (London: Longmans, Brown, and Co., 1857), 50.

68   **deny the existence of a spiritual soul:** Thomas Hobbes, *Leviathan* (1651), paperback ed. (New York: Oxford University Press, 1998), 426.

68   **under experimental control:** Roy Porter, *Flesh in the Age of Reason: The Modern Foundations of Body and Soul* (New York: W. W. Norton, 2003), 91, 93.

68   **called the sweating sickness:** Rosen, *A History of Public Health*, 63–65.

69   **Henry VIII of England:** Porter, *Flesh in the Age of Reason*, 224.

69   **"no small cause":** J. F. Larkin, P. L. Hughes, eds., *Stuart Royal Proclamations, Vol. 1, Royal Proclamations of King James I, 1603–1625* (Oxford: Oxford University Press), cited in Stephen Porter, *The Great Plague* (Phoenix Mill, UK: Sutton, 1999), 17.

69   **half-million by 1660:** Donald R. Hopkins, *The Greatest Killer: Smallpox in History* (Chicago: University of Chicago Press, 2002), 37.

69   **"ten miles off":** Howel and Peter are mentioned by Porter, *The Great Plague*, 19, citing Howel's *Londinopolis* (1658) and Peter's *Good Work for a Good Magistrate* (1651).

69   **[T]he incomparable Aire:** John Evelyn, *The State of France 1652*, published as Appendix B (107–114) in *The Diary of John Evelyn*, vol. 3, E. S. DeBeer, ed. (Oxford: Clarendon, 1955).

70   **"some certain streams":** Daniel Defoe, *A Journal of the Plague Year* (New York: Barnes & Noble Books, 2004), 74–75.

70   **"the wind blowing westward":** William Boghurst, *Loimographia: An Account of the Great Plague of London in Year 1665*, Joseph Frank Payne, ed. (London: Shaw, 1894).

70   **buy some tobacco to smell:** Samuel Pepys, *The Diary of Samuel Pepys*, vol. 6, Robert Latham and William Matthews, eds. (Berkeley: University of California Press, 1972), 120.

70   **had been revivified:** Paul Slack, *The Impact of Plague in Tudor and Stuart England* (Boston: Routledge and Kegan Paul, 1985), 249; Patrick

Wallis, "Plagues, Mortality, and the Place of Medicine in Early Modern England," *English Historical Review* 121, no. 490 (2006): 1–24.

71   **advocacy of "variolation":** Hopkins, *The Greatest Killer*, 10.

71   **those who recover from smallpox:** Ibid., 11.

71   **contagion is propagated:** Richard Mead, *Discourse on the Plague*, 1720 (revised through 1744), cited in *The Medical Works of Dr. Richard Mead*, vol. II (Edinburgh: Donaldson and Reid, 1765), 39, 106.

73   **the subject peoples:** Watts, *Epidemics and History*, 187.

73   **"[T]here is nothing":** John Stuart Mill, *On Liberty* (1859), Currin V. Shields, ed. (Upper Saddle River, NJ: Prentice-Hall, 1997), 14.

73   **Charity, justice, and capital accumulation:** See discussions in Watts, *Epidemics and History*, 186–200; Porter, *Health, Civilization and the State*, 118–125; and Rosen, *A History of Public Health*, 177–197.

73   **ethical, not religious, grounds:** This assessment of Smith and Hume is based on "The Good, the Right, and the Common Point of View," in Simon Blackburn's *Ruling Passions: A Theory of Practical Reasoning* (Oxford: Clarendon, 1998), chap. 7.

73   **never be wholly indifferent to public good:** David Hume, *An Enquiry Concerning the Principles of Morals* (1751), Tom L. Beauchamp, ed. (New York: Oxford University Press, 2006), 75.

73   **commercial and consumerist atmosphere:** Porter, *Flesh in the Age of Reason*, 24.

74   **"intemperate and dissolute":** Rosenberg, *The Cholera Years*, 30, 41–42.

74   **sudden cholera deaths of several prostitutes:** *New York Mercury*, July 18, 1832, cited in Rosenberg, *The Cholera Years*, 42.

74   **higher rates of illness:** Ibid., 59–62.

74   **preference for immigrant-dense towns:** Porter, *Health, Civilization and the State*, 94.

74   **President Zachary Taylor didn't hesitate:** Ibid.; Rosenberg, *The Cholera Years*, 121.

74   **Protestant clergymen responded:** Rosenberg, *The Cholera Years*, 44. Rosenberg mentions F. W. P. Greenwood and the Rev. William Whittingham in particular.

75   **through proper behavior:** The discussion here on cholera and piety in the United States is based on Rosenberg, *The Cholera Years*, chap. 2.

75   **"almost exclusively confined":** John Pintard, *Letters from John Pintard to His Daughter Eliza Noel Pintard Davidson, 1816–1833*, Collections of the New-York Historical Society for the Year 1940, cited in Rosenberg, *The Cholera Years*, 42–43.

75   **American medical men:** Rosenberg, *The Cholera Years*, 76.

75   **"I should not be pained":** Ralph Waldo Emerson, "Man the Reformer," *The Portable Emerson* (New York: Viking Press, 1946), 74–75.

76   **The news that the New York outbreak:** Rosenberg, *The Cholera Years*, 15–16; Geoffrey Marks and William K. Beatty, *Epidemics* (New York: Scribners, 1976), 200–201; John Duffy, *The Sanitarians: A History of American Public Health* (Urbana: University of Illinois Press, 1990), 81.

76   **The German ship:** John C. Peters, "Facts and Theories About the Recent Outbreak of Asiatic Cholera," *New York Medical Journal* 18 (1873): 472–478.

76   **forced by bad weather:** "The Efficacy of Quarantine," *New York Times*, September 25, 1887, 4.

77   **Americans' antipathy toward immigration:** Alan Kraut, *Silent Travelers: Germs, Genes, and the "Immigrant Menace"* (Baltimore: Johns Hopkins University Press, 1994), chap. 2.

77   **1.8 million Irish:** Ibid., 32, citing "The Foreign Immigrant in New York City," a U.S. Industrial Commission report, 1901. The figure for New York residents of Irish descent in 1860 came from a U.S. Census Bureau report not cited by Kraut.

77   **"the miserable outcasts":** *Sunday Times*, March 11, 1849, cited in Rosenberg, *The Cholera Years*, 136.

77   **rumors that cholera:** "Cholera at Niagara," *New York Times*, July 26, 1854, 8.

77   **at least as tolerant of beer drinking:** Rosenberg, *The Cholera Years*, 137–141.

78   **There were 5,017 deaths:** New York City Board of Health, "Report of the Proceedings of the Sanatory Committee," 1849, cited in Rosenberg, *The Cholera Years*, 114. Rosenberg notes that this report shows an increase in deaths attributed to other diarrheal diseases such as dysentery, so some cholera deaths might not have been included in the total, making 5,017 a likely undercount.

78   **the city's population:** Campbell Gibson, "Population of the 100 Largest Cities and Other Urban Places in the United States: 1790 to 1990," U.S. Census Bureau, Table 8 for 1850, at http://www.census.gov/population/documentation/twps0027/tab08.txt (downloaded October 18, 2007).

78   **Americans were complaining:** Newspaper articles of 1849, cited in Rosenberg, *The Cholera Years*, 142.

78   **honest labor in the fresh air:** The argument was first made by Rosenberg, *The Cholera Years*, 150. Georgina Feldberg picks up the idea in her examination of the uses of tuberculosis in shaping the American

middle-class society; see Feldberg, *Disease and Class: Tuberculosis and the Shaping of Modern North American Society* (New Brunswick: Rutgers, 1995), chap. 2.

78   **sand filtration of water supplies:** Rosen, *A History of Public Health*, 130–131.

78   **contamination of drinking water:** Johnson, *The Ghost Map*, 208.

78   **steam pumps to force:** Rosen, *A History of Public Health*, 130.

78   **New York had 105 miles:** Duffy, *The Sanitarians*, 90.

78   **separate systems to pipe:** Rosen, *A History of Public Health*, 130–131.

79   **the link between disease and immigration:** Kraut, *Silent Travelers*, 37–38; Rosenberg, *The Cholera Years*, chap. 10.

80   **impropriety or intemperance:** Rosenberg, *The Cholera Years*, 166.

80   **broader notions about what was good:** Ralph Waldo Emerson asserted as much in his 1836 essay "Nature," writing, "The greatest delight which the fields and woods minister, is the suggestion of an occult relation between man and the vegetable."

80   **I love the forest:** Friedrich Wilhelm Nietzsche, *Thus Spoke Zarathustra: A Book for Everyone and Nobody*, trans. Graham Parkes (New York: Oxford University Press, 2005), 13.

81   ***E. coli* 0157:H7 got into spinach:** U.S. Food and Drug Administration, "Statement on Foodborne E. coli 0157:H7 Outbreak in Spinach," at http://www.fda.gov/bbs/topics/NEWS/2006/NEW01489.html (downloaded October 20, 2007).

81   **the poor neighborhoods of modern-day cities:** See, for instance, Helen Epstein, "The New Ghetto Miasma," *New York Times Magazine*, October 12, 2003.

CHAPTER 4: GERMS, SCIENCE,
AND THE STRANGER

83   **It makes me furious:** Johann Wolfgang von Goethe, *Mephistopheles*, trans. Bayard Taylor (Boston: Houghton Mifflin, 1898).

83   **"more U.S. deaths than AIDS":** "Few U.S. Hospitals Screen Patients for Dangerous Staph 'Superbug,'" Associated Press, October 24, 2007; Winnie Hu and Sarah Kershaw, "Dead Student Had Infection, Officials Say," *New York Times*, October 26, 2007.

83   **SARS burst into the news:** World Health Organization, "Consensus Document on the Severe Acute Respiratory Syndrome (SARS)," 2003, at http://w.who.int/csr/rsnHOconsensus.pdf (downloaded October 27, 2007); D. L. Heyman and G. Rodier, "Global Surveillance, National Surveillance, and SARS," *Emerging Infectious Diseases*, February 2003,

at http://www.cdc.gov/ncidod/EID/v0110n02/03-1038.htm (down-loaded October 27, 2007).

84   **8,098 cases and 774 deaths:** World Health Organization, "Summary of Probable SARS Cases With Onset of Illness from 1 November 2002 to 31 July 2003," at http://www.who.int/csr/sars/country/table2003_09 _23/en/ (downloaded October 27, 2007).

84   **"first epidemic of the twenty-first century":** Tim Brookes and Omar A. Khan, *Behind the Mask: How the World Survived SARS, the First Epidemic of the 21st Century* (Washington, DC: American Public Health Association, 2005).

84   **thermal-scanning procedures:** D. M. Bell and WHO Working Group on Prevention of International and Community Transmission of SARS, "Public Health Interventions and SARS Spread," *Emerging Infectious Diseases* 10, no. 11 (2004): 1900–1906.

84   **Officials asked 3,000 people:** Denise Grady, "Fear Reigns as Dangerous Mystery Illness Spreads," *New York Times*, April 7, 2003.

85   **"jet-borne killer disease":** Bernard Orsman, "NZ Joins Watch for Jet-Borne Killer Disease," *New Zealand Herald*, March 17, 2003.

85   **"first jet-set plague":** Michael Hanlon, "SARS, the World's First Jet-Set Plague," *Daily Mail* (London), April 22, 2003.

85   **simply as the "super-bug":** Anna Patty, "Super-Bug Alert," *Advertiser* (Australia), March 19, 2003.

85   **"The New Plague":** Amy Harmon, "Public Confronts New Virus on Laymen's Terms," *New York Times*, April 6, 2003.

85   **Plans for bioterrorism response:** Paul H. B. Shin, "City's Rushing to Slam Door on SARS: Using Bioterror Plans to Combat Deadly Virus," *Daily News* (NY), April 25, 2003.

85   **Rolling Stones:** Gayle MacDonald and James Adams, "Stones Cancel Hong Kong Concerts," *Globe and Mail*, March 28, 2003.

85   **Morgan Stanley:** Denise Grady, "Fear Reigns as Dangerous Mystery Illness Spreads," *New York Times*, April 7, 2003.

86   **"aerosolizing incidents":** WHO, "Consensus Document," 24.

86   **"superspreaders":** Stefan Lovgren, "The Mystery of the SARS Virus: How Is It Spread?" *National Geographic News*, April 9, 2003, at http://news.nationalgeographic.com/news/2003/04/0409_030409_sars .html (downloaded October 28, 2007); Hannah Beech, "Doing Battle with the Bug," *Time*, April 7, 2003; "superspreaders" were also the subject of four *New York Times* articles, a story on the Canadian Broadcasting System, and a CNN piece.

86   **quarantine camp:** Erik Eckholm, "Beijing Broadens SARS Quarantine, More Cases Found," *New York Times*, April 26, 2003.

86 entire dormitories: Michael Jen-Siu and Bill Savadove, "Beijing Virus Fight Sees Thousands Shut In," *South China Morning Post* (Hong Kong), April 26, 2003.

86 1.7 million Beijing children: John Pomfret, "Schools Are Closed as Toll in Capital Rises to 35 Dead," *Washington Post*, April 24, 2003.

86 Two thousand patients: Joseph Kahn, "Quarantine Set in Beijing Areas to Fight SARS," *New York Times*, April 23, 2003.

86 Another 2,000: Eckholm, "Beijing Broadens SARS Quarantine."

86 Thousands fled: Pomfret, "Schools Are Closed."

87 "forbidden to enter": Erik Eckholm, "With Virus at the Gate, the Drawbridge Is Up," *New York Times*, April 28, 2003.

87 vigilantes standing with bottles of disinfectant: "Village Riots in Fear of Virus," *Herald Sun* (Melbourne), April 30, 2003.

87 banks sterilized banknotes: Ibid.

87 taxi drivers refused: Joseph Kahn and Elizabeth Rosenthal, "Even in Remote China, SARS Arrives in Force," *International Herald Tribune*, April 23, 2003.

87 travel permits: Kahn, "Quarantine Set in Beijing Areas to Fight SARS."

87 284 patients and staff: Annie Freeda Cruez, "284 Quarantined at Kuching Mental Hospital," *New Straits Times* (Malaysia), April 28, 2003.

87 sporadic fatalities: WHO, "Summary of Probable SARS Cases with Onset of Illness from 1 November 2002 to 31 July 2003," September 26, 2003, at http://www.who.int/csr/sars/country/table2003_09_23/en/ (downloaded December 8, 2008).

89 accounts of AIDS: Randy Shilts, *And the Band Played On* (New York: Penguin, 1988), 3; Laurie Garrett, *The Coming Plague* (New York: Penguin, 1995), 263.

92 the February Revolution: R. J. W. Evans and Hartmut Pogge von Strandmann, eds., *The Revolutions in Europe, 1848–1849: From Reform to Reaction* (Oxford: Oxford University Press, 2000).

92 Epidemiology, the study of epidemic illness: The word "epidemiology" first appeared in an 1802 treatise by Don Joaquin Villalba recounting epidemics that had struck the Iberian Peninsula, called *Epidemiología Española.*

92 seminal article on epidemiology: Louis-René Villermé, "De la mortalité dans divers quartiers de la ville de Paris," *Annales d'hygiene publique* 3 (1830): 294–341.

93 poverty was the impediment: Material on Villermé and the *partie d'hygiene* based on Dorothy Porter, *Health, Civilization and the State: A History of Public Health from Ancient to Modern Times* (New York: Routledge, 1999), 68–69.

93   **"radical action":** Here is Virchow's observation on the effectiveness of
the Prussian state, so proud of its organizing capacity, once typhus
came: "The law existed, the civil servants were there—and the people
died in their thousands from starvation and disease. The law did not
help, as it was only paper with writing; the civil servants did no good,
for the result of their activity again was only writing on paper. . . . The
bureaucracy would not, or could not, help the people. . . . The plutoc-
racy did not recognize the Upper Silesians as human beings, but only as
tools. . . . The clerical hierarchy endorsed the wretched neediness of
the people as a ticket to heaven." Rudolf Virchow, "Report on the Typhus Epidemic in Upper Silesia," *Archiv für pathologische Anatomie und
Physiologie und für klinische Medicin*, excerpted in *American Journal of
Public Health* 96, no. 12 (2006): 2102–2105, from L. J. Rather, ed., *Collected Essays in Public Health and Epidemiology*, vol. 1 (Boston: Science
History Publications, 1985).

93   **social remediation:** George Rosen, *A History of Public Health*, expanded ed. (Baltimore: Johns Hopkins, 1993), 232.

94   **scientific studies of causes and conditions:** Ralph Frerichs, London
Epidemiological Society Web site, at http://www.ph.ucla.edu/EPI/
snow/LESociety.html (downloaded December 7, 2008).

94   **"combated and expelled":** Alun Evans, "Benjamin Guy Babington:
Founding President of the London Epidemiological Society," *International Journal of Epidemiology* 30 (2001): 226–230.

94   **Statistik:** Gottfried Achenwall, *Vorbereitung zur Staatswissenschaft der
heutigen fürnehmsten Europäischen Reiche und Staaten* (Göttingen: Van-
denhoeck, 1748).

95   **social reform:** Porter, *Health, Civilization and the State*, 72.

95   **committees on smallpox:** Warren Winkelstein Jr., "Interface of Epidemiology and History: A Commentary on Past, Present, and Future,"
Epidemiologic Reviews 22, no. 1 (2000): 2–6.

96   **social as well as biological:** Porter, *Health, Civilization and the State*, 84.

96   **considerable opposition:** Rosen, *A History of Public Health*, 277.

96   **commercial expansion:** Porter, *Health, Civilization and the State*, 82–83.

96   **electrical theory involving ozone:** Steven Johnson, *The Ghost Map*
(New York: Penguin, 2007), 122–123.

97   **Anti-contagionist arguments:** Rosen, *A History of Public Health*, 266;
Sheldon Watts, *Epidemics and History: Disease, Power, and Imperialism*
(New Haven: Yale University Press, 1997), 194.

97   **driven by impropriety:** Georgina Feldberg, *Disease and Class: Tuberculosis and the Shaping of Modern North American Society* (New Brunswick:
Rutgers University Press, 1995).

97   **asserting that cholera was a type of fever:** Watts, *Epidemics and History*, 193.

97   **"parent of disease":** D. Francis Condie, *All the Material Facts in the History of Epidemic Cholera* (Philadelphia, 1832), quoted in Charles E. Rosenberg, *The Cholera Years* (Chicago: University of Chicago Press, 1962), 56. See, more generally, Rosenberg, *The Cholera Years*, chaps. 2 and 3.

98   **embrace laboratory science:** Paul Starr, *The Social Transformation of American Medicine* (New York: Basic Books, 1982), chaps. 2 and 3; Roy Porter, *Bodies Politic: Disease, Death and Doctors in Britain, 1650–1900* (Ithaca: Cornell University Press, 2001).

98   **new weaponry:** Michael Howard, *The Franco-Prussian War: The German Invasion of France, 1870–1871* (New York: Routledge, 2001).

98   **circumstances of life:** Roy Porter, *Flesh in the Age of Reason: The Modern Foundations of Body and Soul* (New York: W. W. Norton, 2004), 418.

98   **A signal event:** Material in this paragraph is based on the account by Rosen, *A History of Public Health*, 280–291.

99   **different bacteria:** Ibid., 290.

99   **so-called carriers:** Ibid., 295–296.

100   **perfection of humankind:** Mark Francis, *Herbert Spencer and the Invention of Modern Life* (Ithaca: Cornell University Press, 2007).

100   **Haeckel went further:** Ernst Klee, *"Euthanasie" im NS-Staat: Die "Vernichtung Lebensunwerten Lebens."* (Frankfurt: Fischer, 1985), 16.

101   **culling the unfit:** John B. Haycraft, "Natural Selection and Race Improvement," cited in Klee, *Euthanasie*, 17.

102   **recent scientific report:** J. Gudmundsson, P. Sulem, A. Manolescu, L. T. Amundadottir et al., "Genome-Wide Association Study Identifies a Second Prostate Cancer Susceptibility Variant at 8q24," *Nature Genetics* 39 (2007): 631–637.

102   **recent article in a peer-reviewed epidemiology journal:** D. K. Eaton, L. Kann, S. Kinchen, J. Ross, et al. "Youth Risk Behavior Surveillance—United States, 2005," *Morbidity and Mortality Weekly Report Surveillance Summaries* 55, no. SS05 (June 9, 2006): 1–108.

103   **"seed and soil":** See Feldberg, *Disease and Class*, chap. 2 for an insightful discussion of the seed-and-soil belief and its consequences.

103   **It was predisposition:** Ibid.; Nancy Tomes, *The Gospel of Germs: Men, Women, and the Microbe in American Life* (Cambridge: Harvard University Press, 1998), 46.

103   **"congenial soil":** L. Bremer, "The Bearing of the Discovery of the Tubercle Bacillus on Public Hygiene," *St. Louis Medical and Surgical Journal* 47 (1884): 496, cited in Feldberg, *Disease and Class*, 46.

103   **TB is caused by:** August Flint and William H. Welch, *The Principles and Practice of Medicine*, 5th ed., 1881, cited in Susan Sontag, *Illness as Metaphor and AIDS and its Metaphors* (New York: Anchor/Doubleday, 1990), 54.

104   **"far too one-sided":** H. F. Formad, "The Bacillus Tuberulosis and the Etiology of Tuberculosis," *Philadelphia Medical Times* 14 (1883–1884): 337–338, cited in Feldberg, *Disease and Class*, 43.

104   **he warned that "associated influences":** E. Hunt, "Hygiene and Its Scope, Its Progress and Its Leading Aims," address to the American Public Health Association meeting, 1883, cited in Feldberg, *Disease and Class*, 45.

105   **The nativist movement:** This paragraph is based on the historical accounts by Alan M. Kraut, *Silent Travelers: Germs, Genes, and the Immigrant Menace* (Baltimore: Johns Hopkins, 1994), chaps. 3–7; Howard Markel, *Quarantine! East European Jewish Immigrants and the New York City Epidemics of 1892* (Baltimore: Johns Hopkins University Press, 1997), chap. 1; and Markel, *When Germs Travel: Six Major Epidemics That Invaded America Since 1900 and the Fears They Unleashed* (New York: Pantheon, 2004).

105   **Chinese people harbored:** Arthur B. Stout, "Report on Chinese Immigration," 1870–1871, cited in Kraut, *Silent Travelers*, 81.

106   **Intensive medical inspections:** Markel, *Quarantine!* chap. 1; Markel, "'The Eyes Have It': Trachoma, the Perception of Disease, the United States Public Health Service, and the American Jewish Immigration Experience, 1897–1924," *Bulletin of the History of Medicine* 74, no. 3 (2000): 525–560; Markel, *When Germs Travel*; Kraut, *Silent Travelers*, chap. 3.

106   **less likely to die of polio:** Kraut, *Silent Travelers*, 108, 126–128.

106   **50 percent less likely than native-born citizens:** Louis I. Dublin and Gladden W. Baker, "The Mortality of Race Stocks in Pennsylvania and New York," *Quarterly Publication of the American Statistical Association*, 17, no. 129 (March 1920): 13–44.

106   **implication and immunity:** This opposition of "implicated" and "immune" was proposed by Richard Goldstein in regard to AIDS. See "A Disease of Society: Cultural Responses to AIDS," *The Milbank Quarterly*, vol. 68, supplement 2, part 2 (1990): 295–319.

107   **engines of degradation:** Markel, *Quarantine!* 35–36, 146–152.

107   **In 1900, an outbreak of plague:** The details of the plague outbreak in San Franciso in 1900 and the political response it elicited are given by Kraut, *Silent Travelers*, chap. 4; and Marilyn Chase, *The Barbary Plague: The Black Death in Victorian San Francisco* (New York: Random House, 2003).

108   impermissible to quarantine: *Jew Ho v. Williamson*, 103 F. 10 (CCND Cal. 1900).

108   infected wealthy Americans: Judith Walzer Leavitt, *Typhoid Mary: Captive to the Public's Health* (Boston: Beacon Press, 1996).

108   By about 1910, germs had been shown: Rosen, *A History of Public Health*, 303.

109   expression of character: This is one of the themes of Sontag's *Illness as Metaphor and AIDS and its Metaphors*.

109   antisepsis and then sterilization made hospitals look clean: Rosen, *A History of Public Health*, 292–294; Tomes, *The Gospel of Germs*, 103–104.

109   Special fears of dust and dirt: Tomes, *The Gospel of Germs*, 96–97.

109   the true number of casualties is unknown: N. P. Johnson and J. Mueller, "Updating the Accounts: Global Mortality of the 1918–1920 'Spanish' Influenza Pandemic," *Bulletin of the History of Medicine* 76, no. 1 (Spring 2002): 105–115; Jeffery K. Taubenberger and David M. Morens, "1918 Influenza: The Mother of All Pandemics," *Emerging Infectious Diseases* 12, no. 1 (January 2006): 15–22.

110   somewhat lower mortality rates: H. Markel, H. B. Lipman, A. Navarro, et al., "Nonpharmaceutical Interventions Implemented by US Cities During the 1918–1919 Influenza Pandemic," *JAMA* 298 (2007): 644–654.

110   W-shaped pattern of mortality: P. Palese, "Influenza: Old and New Threats," *Nature Medicine* 12, no. 10 (2004): 582–587; Taubenberger and Morens, "1918 Influenza," 19–20.

110   labeled "Spanish": This explanation appears in John M. Barry, *The Great Influenza: The Epic Story of the Deadliest Plague in History* (New York: Viking, 2004), 171. I have found no more compelling explanation for the name "Spanish Flu."

111   first mentioned in New York papers: "Spanish Influenza Here, Ship Men Say; Officers of Norwegian Liner Attribute Four Deaths During Voyage to the Disease," *New York Times*, August 14, 1918.

111   poor ventilation: R. Tellier, "Review of Aerosol Transmission of Influenza A Virus," *Emerging Infectious Diseases* 12, no. 11 (2006): 1657–1662.

111   banning large gatherings: Howard Markel, Alexandra M. Stern, J. Alexander Navarro, et al., "Nonpharmaceutical Influenza Mitigation Strategies, US Communities, 1918–1920 Pandemic," *Emerging Infectious Diseases* 12, no. 12 (December 2006), at http://wwwdc.gov/ncidod/eid/vol12no12/06-0506.htm (downloaded December 7, 2008).

111   "Garden of Germs": Naomi Rogers, *Dirt and Disease: Polio Before FDR* (New Brunswick: Rutgers, 1996), 9.

112   **America's midsection:** Evidence that the pandemic virus strain originated in Haskell County, Kansas, is summarized in Barry, *The Great Influenza*, chaps. 6 and 7.

112   **the swine flu affair:** Detailed in Richard E. Neustadt and Harvey V. Fineberg, *The Swine Flu Affair: Decision-Making on a Slippery Disease* (U.S. Department of Health, Education and Welfare, 1978).

112   **45 million Americans had been immunized:** Walter Dowdle, "The 1976 Experience," *Journal of Infectious Diseases* 176, suppl. 1 (1997): S69–S72.

112   **$93 million:** Garrett, *The Coming Plague*, 182.

112   **human cases began to appear in China:** Data from World Health Organization, "H5N1 Avian Influenza: Timeline of Major Events," at http://www.who.int/csr/disease/avian_influenza/Timeline_17_Dec_07.pdf (downloaded December 7, 2008).

113   **more than 380 human cases:** World Health Organization, "Epidemic and Pandemic Alert and Response: Avian Flu," at http://www.who.int/csr/disease/avian_influenza/country/cases_table_2008_09_10/en/index.html (downloaded December 7, 2008).

113   **not infected at high rates:** Sirenda Vong, Benjamin Coghlan, Sek Mardy, Davun Holl, et al., "Low Frequency of Poultry-to-Human H5N1 Virus Transmission, Southern Cambodia, 2005," *Emerging Infectious Diseases* 12, no. 10 (October 2006): 1542–1547.

113   **migratory birds are not very susceptible:** Justin D. Brown, David E. Stallknecht, Joan R. Beck, David L. Suarez, and David E. Swayne, "Susceptibility of North American Ducks and Gulls to H5N1 Highly Pathogenic Avian Influenza Viruses," *Emerging Infectious Diseases* 12, no. 11 (2006): 1663–1670.

113   **scientists and officials have invoked the Spanish Flu scenario:** For instance, R. G. Webster, M. Peiris, H. Chen, and Y. Guan, "H5N1 Outbreaks and Enzootic Influenza," *Emerging Infectious Diseases* 12 (2006): 3–8; U.S. Centers for Disease Control and Prevention, "Avian Flu: Current H5N1 Situation," at http://www.cdc.gov/flu/avian/outbreaks/current.htm (downloaded December 7, 2008); U.S. Department of Health and Human Services, "Community Strategy for Pandemic Influenza Mitigation" at http://www.pandemicflu.gov/plan/community/commitigation.html (downloaded December 8, 2008); Mike Davis, "Avian Flu: A State of Unreadiness" *Nation* (July 18–25, 2005): 27–30.

113   **elegant scientific work:** T. M. Tumpey, C. F. Basler, P. V. Aguilar, H. Zeng, et al., "Characterization of the Reconstructed 1918 Spanish Influenza Pandemic Virus," *Science* 310 (2005): 77–80; J. K. Taubenberger,

A. H. Reid, R. M. Lourens, R. Wang et al., "Characterization of the 1918 Influenza Virus Polymerase Genes. *Nature* 437 (2005): 887–893.

113   **such resistance exists in China:** K. F. Shortridge, "Pandemic Influenza: A Zoonosis?" *Seminars in Respiratory Infection* 7 (1992): 11–25.

117   **"web of causation":** B. MacMahon and T. F. Pugh, *Epidemology: Principles and Methods* (Boston: Little, Brown, 1970), 23–25.

117   **interacting systems:** M. Susser and E. Susser, "Choosing a Future for Epidemiology: I. Eras and Paradigms," *American Journal of Public Health* 86 (1996): 668–673; M. Susser and E. Susser, "Choosing a Future for Epidemiology: II. From Black Box to Chinese Boxes and Eco-Epidemiology," *American Journal of Public Health* 86 (1996): 674–677.

117   **what happens in science:** For the full critique of Kuhn, and the curious relation of Kuhn's theory to developments in biological science, see Steve Fuller, *Kuhn vs. Popper: The Struggle for the Soul of Science* (New York: Columbia University Press, 2004), 46–48.

CHAPTER 5: THE CONQUEST OF CONTAGION

119   **A tropical entropy seemed to prevail:** Joan Didion, *Miami* (New York: Vintage, 1998), 27–28.

119   **so-called first responders:** The updated version of the CDC announcement, including the president's plan, can be seen at the CDC Web site. See "Protecting Americans: Smallpox Vaccination Program," at http://www.bt.cdc.gov/agent/smallpox/vaccination/vaccination-program-statement.asp, (downloaded December 10, 2008).

119   **Bush announced:** "Smallpox Vaccination: Implementation of National Program Faces Challenges," General Accounting Office, April 2003, at http://www.gao.gov/new.items/d03578.pdf (downloaded November 27, 2006).

120   **"the plague bacillus":** Albert Camus, *The Plague*, trans. Stuart Gilbert (New York: Vintage, 1991), 308.

121   **Syphilis swept through Europe:** William H. McNeill, *Plagues and Peoples* (New York: Anchor/Doubleday, 1977), 157, 193.

122   **the neonatal death rate:** J. T. Biggs, "Sanitation vs. Vaccination, 1912," at http://www.whale.to/a/biggs_b.html (downloaded December 14, 2007).

122   **2 percent of U.S. servicemen:** "Report of the Surgeon General of the U.S. Army, 1910" (USGPO, 1911), cited in Allan Brandt, *No Magic Bullet: A Social History of Venereal Disease in the United States Since 1880* (New York: Oxford University Press, 1985), 13.

122   **10 percent of all Americans:** John H. Stokes, *The Third Great Plague: A Discussion of Syphilis for Everyday People* (Philadelphia: W. B. Saun-

ders, 1920), 26, cited in Nicolas Jabbour, "Syphilis from 1880 to 1920: A Public Health Nightmare and the First Challenge to Medical Ethics," *Essays in History* 42 (2000), at http://etext.virginia.edu/journals/EH/EH42/Jabbour42.html (downloaded January 12, 2009).

122   **Progressives responded by working:** Kristin Luker, *When Sex Goes to School: Warring Views on Sex—and Sex Education—Since the Sixties* (New York: W. W. Norton, 2006), 37.

123   **they thought the working classes:** Brandt, *No Magic Bullet*, 29.

123   **marriage would be promoted:** Luker, *When Sex Goes to School*, 45–62.

123   **future generations:** Brandt, *No Magic Bullet*, 27. Material in this and subsequent paragraphs from pp. 17–27.

123   **social-hygiene campaign took the form:** The story of the first sexual revolution is told by Luker, *When Sex Goes to School*, chap. 2, and by Brandt, *No Magic Bullet*, chap. 1. Details on industry and advertising in the war against germs are given by Nancy Tomes, *The Gospel of Germs: Men, Women, and the Microbe in American Life* (Cambridge: Harvard University Press, 1998), chap. 7.

124   **suppressed sex work:** This is a main theme of Brandt's discussion of the history of venereal disease in America in *No Magic Bullet*.

124   **the modernization of manufacturing:** Ibid., 34. Brandt attributes these claims to vice commissions in New York and Chicago.

125   **bring home VD:** Ibid., illustrations following 110.

125   **posters and training films:** Examples of these posters are found in ibid. and in "Visual Culture and Public Health Posters: Venereal Disease," an online exhibit by the National Library of Medicine, September 2003, at http://www.nlm.nih.gov/exhibition/visualculture/venereal.html (downloaded December 20, 2007).

125   **American purity crusaders sought continence:** Brandt, *No Magic Bullet*, 35–40.

126   **"Secretly I don't believe":** Cited in Susan Sontag, *Illness as Metaphor and AIDS and its Metaphors* (New York: Anchor/Doubleday, 1990), 44.

126   **Syphilis and gonorrhea were brought under some control:** Centers for Disease Control, "Achievements in Public Health, 1900–1999: Control of Infectious Diseases," *Morbidity and Mortality Weekly Report* 48, no. 29 (July 30, 1999): 621–628. New-case rates for both syphilis and gonorrhea declined dramatically through the 1950s, as evident in a U.S. Public Health Service graph, "Cases of Venereal Disease Reported by State Health Departments, and Rates Per 100,000 Population," reproduced in Brandt, *No Magic Bullet*, appendix.

126   **more of an evolution:** Alfred E. Kinsey, et al., *Sexual Behavior in the Human Male* (Philadelphia: W. B. Saunders, 1948); Morton Hunt, *Sexual*

Behavior in the 1970s (Chicago: Playboy Press, 1974); Jeffrey Weeks, *Sex, Politics and Society: The Regulation of Sex since 1800* (London: Longman, 1981), all cited in Brandt, *No Magic Bullet*, 175.

127 **control declined:** Brandt, *No Magic Bullet*, 178.

127 **exchanged sex for either money or drugs:** Centers for Disease Control, "Relationship of Syphilis to Drug and Prostitution—Connecticut and Philadelphia, Pennsylvania," *Morbidity and Mortality Weekly Report* 37, no. 49 (December 16, 1988): 755–758, 764; also CDC, Epidemiologic Notes and Reports: Multiple Strain Outbreak of Penicillinase-Producing Neisseria Gonorrhoeae—Denver, Colorado, 1986," *Morbidity and Mortality Weekly Report* 36, no. 32 (August 21, 1987): 534–536, 542–543; also further reports in the 1990s. Archived *MMWR* reports are accessible at http://www.cdc.gov/mmwr/mmwrpvol.html.

128 **"pack of children":** Robert Boyce, "The Colonization of Africa," *Journal of the African Society* 10, no. 40 (1911): 394–396, quoted in Sheldon Watts, *Epidemics and History: Disease, Power, and Imperialism* (New Haven: Yale University Press, 1997), 258.

128 **"the native":** Ronald Ross, quoted in Watts, *Epidemics and History*, 256.

128 **"colonial medicine":** Maryinez Lyons, *The Colonial Disease: A Social History of Sleeping Sickness in Northern Zaire, 1900–1940* (New York: Cambridge University Press, 1992), 69.

129 **low frequency of yellow fever:** Watts, *Epidemics and History*, 217, quoting W. H. Hoffman, "Yellow Fever in Africa from the Epidemiological Standpoint," in M. B. Khalil, ed., Proceedings, Congrès International de Médecine Tropicale et d'Hygiène, Cairo, Egypt, Govt. Printing Office, 1928.

129 **"you cannot have omelettes":** Quoted in Watts, *Epidemics and History*, 261.

129 **Ziel und Weg:** Robert Proctor, *Racial Hygiene: Medicine Under the Nazis* (Cambridge: Harvard University Press, 1988), 24, 65.

129 **In France, medical authorities:** Ibid., 159.

130 **forcibly sterilized people:** Robert Jay Lifton, *The Nazi Doctors: Medical Killing and the Psychology of Genocide* (New York: Perseus, 1986), 25.

130 **excuse to sterilize perpetrators of "sex crimes":** Robert Proctor, *Racial Hygiene: Medicine Under the Nazis* (Cambridge: Harvard University Press, 1988), 77; James M. Glass, *"Life Unworthy of Life": Racial Phobia and Mass Murder in Hitler's Germany* (New York: Basic Books, 1997), 40. The text of the law was translated into English by the Cold Spring Harbor Eugenics Lab and published in *Eugenics News* 18, no. 5 (1933), at http://www.eugenicsarchive.org/html/eugenics/index2.html ?tag=1901 (downloaded October 11, 2008).

130   **"It is better for all":** Material in this paragraph from Harry Bruinius, *Better for All the World: The Secret History of Forced Sterilization and America's Quest for Racial Purity* (New York: Knopf, 2006), 17, 57–58, 71–72.

131   **honorary doctorate:** Stephen H. Norwood, "Harvard's Nazi Ties," David S. Wyman Institute for Holocaust Studies, November 2004, at http://www.wymaninstitute.org/articles/2004-11-harvard.php (downloaded January 17, 2008).

131   **Dr. H. E. Kleinschmidt:** W. W. Peter, "Germany's Sterilization Program," *American Journal of Public Health* 24 (1934): 187–191; H. E. Kleinschmidt, "New Germany Teaches Her People: An Account of the Health Exposition in Berlin," *American Journal of Public Health* 25 (1935): 1108–1113. See also Glass, "Life Unworthy of Life," 44–46.

131   **"the anti-Semitic policy":** Kleinschmidt, "New Germany Teaches," 1111.

131   **T4 had exterminated 70,273 Germans:** Götz Aly, Peter Chroust, and Christian Pross, *Cleansing the Fatherland: Nazi Medicine and Racial Hygiene* (Baltimore: Johns Hopkins, 1994), 39. Material in this and following two paragraphs on Nazi euthanasia is drawn from Chapter 2.

132   **Poles who had tuberculosis:** Lifton, *The Nazi Doctors*, 136.

132   **"when diseased":** Cited in Harriett Washington, *Medical Apartheid: The Dark History of Medical Experimentation on Black Americans from Colonial Times to the Present* (New York: Doubleday, 2006), 157.

133   **at higher risk:** See, for example, the Office for Minority Health and Health Disparities at the U.S. Centers for Disease Control and Prevention, at http://www.cdc.gov/omhd/Populations/BAA/BAA.htm#Disparities (downloaded on December 12, 2008).

133   **prostate cancer:** U.S. National Center for Health Statistics (NCHS), "Health, United States, 2007," Age-adjusted cancer incidence rates for selected cancer sites, by sex, race, and Hispanic origin: United States, selected geographic areas, selected years, 1990–2004, table 53, at http://www.cdc.gov/nchs/hus.htm (downloaded December 12, 2008).

133   **hepatitis B virus:** C. Marwick, M. Mitka, "Debate Revived on Hepatitis B Vaccine Value," *JAMA* 282, no. 1 (1999): 15–17.

133   **HIV:** NCHS, "Health, United States, 2007," tables 42 and 52, at http://www.cdc.gov/nchs/hus.htm (downloaded December 12, 2008).

133   **infant mortality:** G. K. Singh and S. M. Yu, "Infant Mortality in the United States: Trends, Differentials, and Projections, 1950 through 2010," *American Journal of Public Health* 85 (1995): 957–964.

133   **"where rats appear":** Julius H. Schoeps, "Kein Führerbefehl zum Mord," *Die Zeit*, November 1986, at http://zeus.zeit.de/text/1986/11/Zt19860307 _023_0031_Pol (downloaded December 17, 2007). Images and text

available at the Holocaust History Project Web site, at http://www
.holocaust-history.org/der-ewige-jude/stills.shtml (downloaded December 12, 2008).

133   a *Pestherd:* Ian Kershaw, *Hitler, 1936–1945: Nemesis* (New York: W. W. Norton, 2000). Kershaw gives the Hitler quote, translating Hitler's word *Pestherd* as "plague center." Hitler's reference was to Russia's large Jewish population. "Plague focus" seems a slightly better translation; Hitler was alluding to the medical term "focus of infection," from which bacterial infection might later become widespread or, in medical parlance, "systemic." Thus, Hitler's remark, made in July 1941, very shortly after Germany broke its 1939 pact with the Soviet Union and invaded its former ally, portrayed Russia as not merely nefarious but noxious to Western Europe. In *Masters of Death: The SS-Einsatzgruppen and the Invention of the Holocaust* (New York: Knopf, 2002), Richard Rhodes notes that Hitler made the statement to the Slovakian minister of defense, just at the point when Heinrich Himmler, who had been given authority over civil administration in Nazi-occupied territories in Eastern Europe, was ordering the Final Solution for Jews in the eastern occupied territories.

134   **"as we exterminate the bacillus":** A recording and partial transcription are available at the Holocaust History Project Web site, http://www.holocaust
-history.org/himmler-poznan/ (downloaded December 12, 2008).

135   **Few clinics were open to black residents:** Charles S. Johnson, *Shadow of the Plantation* (Chicago: University of Chicago Press, 1934), 186–207. Descriptions of medical conditions and care in Macon County, Alabama, are reprinted in Susan M. Reverby, ed., *Tuskegee's Truths: Rethinking the Tuskegee Syphilis Study* (Chapel Hill: University of North Carolina Press, 2000), 41 ff.

135   **36 percent of residents:** James Jones, *Bad Blood: The Tuskegee Syphilis Experiment,* expanded ed. (New York: Free Press, 1993), 27, 74.

135   **men under observation:** Ibid., 177–179.

135   **untreated syphilis in men:** The findings were based on a retrospective review of cases in Oslo, Norway, of men who for one reason or another had not received the partially effective treatment with arsenic derivatives. See T. Gjestland, "The Oslo Study of Untreated Syphilis: An Epidemiologic Investigation of the Boeck-Bruusgaard Material," *Acta Derm Venereol* 35, supplement 34 (1955): 1; also E. G. Clark and N. Danbolt, "The Oslo Study of the Natural Course of Untreated Syphilis: An Epidemiologic Investigation Based on a Re-study of the Boeck-Bruusgaard Material," *Medical Clinics of North America* 48 (1964): 613–623.

135   **committed against the disfavored:** Washington, *Medical Apartheid.*

135   **without "equipose":** The notion that research is justified when scientists are in the state of equipoise, i.e., of not knowing which of two alternative explanations is correct, has been much exploited, as Tuskegee demonstrates. For attempts at rationalizing research based on equipoise, see B. Freedman, "Equipoise and the Ethics of Clinical Research," *New England Journal of Medicine* 317 (1987): 141–145; C. Weijer and E. J. Emanuel, "Protecting Communities in Biomedical Research," *Science* 289 (2000): 1142–1144; and C. Weijer, S. H. Shapiro, K. C. Glass, "Clinical Equipoise and not the Uncertainty Principle Is the Moral Underpinning of the Randomized Controlled Trial," *British Medical Journal* 321 (2000): 756–758.

136   **"end of the negro problem":** Thomas Murrell, "Syphilis and the American Negro: A Medico-Sociological Study," *JAMA* 54 (1910): 846–847, cited in Washington, *Medical Apartheid*, 160.

136   **insisted either that brothels be opened:** George Walker, *Venereal Disease in the American Expeditionary Force* (Baltimore: Medical Standard Book Co., 1922), cited in Brandt, *No Magic Bullet*, 104.

137   **order immediate sterilization:** Washington, *Medical Apartheid*, 194. Washington summarizes the evidence, citing in particular an article by Robert W. Kesting, "Blacks Under the Swastika, a Research Note," *Journal of Negro History* 83, no. 1 (1998): 84–99.

137   **ruin the well-bred family:** The canonical work on Haiselden is Martin S. Pernick, *The Black Stork: Eugenics and the Death of "Defective" Babies in American Medicine and Motion Pictures since 1915* (New York: Oxford University Press, 1999).

137   **The American eugenics movement:** Edwin Black, *War Against the Weak: Eugenics and America's Campaign to Create a Master Race* (New York: Four Walls Eight Windows, 2003), chap. 20.

137   **generalized distaste:** Ibid., chap. 15.

138   **more than 5,000 deaths:** A. B. Bloch, W. A. Orenstein, H. C. Stetler, et al., "Health Impact of Measles Vaccination in the United States," *Pediatrics* 76, no. 4 (1985): 524–532.

141   **germ theory gave the study of epidemics:** For this examination of historicity I draw on the argument advanced by Steve Fuller in *Kuhn vs. Popper: The Struggle for the Soul of Modern Science* (New York: Columbia University Press, 2004).

141   **successive shifts in thought:** Framing the processes of the science industry as essentially anarchic, leaving truth to be claimed by the most powerful or the craftiest, is the argument made by Paul Feyerabend in *Against Method: Outline of an Anarchistic Theory of Knowledge*, revised ed. (San Francisco: Analytical Psychology Club, 1988).

142   **his 1943 history:** Charles-Edward Amory Winslow, *The Conquest of Epidemic Disease: A Chapter in the History of Ideas* (Princeton: Princeton University Press, 1943).

142   **"victory" over polio:** "Polio Conquered," *Chicago Daily Tribune*, April 13, 1955; "Conquest of Polio," *Los Angles Times*, April 13, 1955.

CHAPTER 6: POSTMODERN EPIDEMICS

143   **Whenever an evil:** Friedrich Nietzsche, *Daybreak (Die Morgenröte)* (1881), book 1, no. 33, eds. Maudemarie Clark and Brian Leiter, trans. R. J. Hollingdale (Cambridge: Cambridge, 1997), 24.

144   **hypothesizing that a toxin elaborated:** J. Todd, M. Fishaut, F. Kapral, and T. Welch, "Toxic-Shock Syndrome Associated with Phage-Group I Staphylococci," *Lancet 2*, (1978): 1116–1118.

144   **three similar cases appeared among Wisconsin women:** J. P. Davis, J. Chesney, P. J. Wand, et al., "Toxic-Shock Syndrome," *New England Journal of Medicine* 303 (1980): 1429–1435.

144   **fifty-five cases had been reported:** Centers for Disease Control (CDC), "Toxic-Shock Syndrome—United States," *Morbidity and Mortality Weekly Report* 29 (1980): 229–230.

144   **the CDC asserted:** CDC, "Follow-up on Toxic-Shock Syndrome—United States," *Morbidity and Mortality Weekly Report* 29, no. 20 (1980): 297–299.

144   **statistical association:** CDC. "Follow-up on Toxic-Shock Syndrome," *Morbidity and Mortality Weekly Report* 29, no. 37 (1980): 441–445.

144   **discourage a product's use:** U.S. Food & Drug Administration news release PBD-42, September 25, 1980, cited in Laurie Garrett, *The Coming Plague: Newly Emerging Diseases in a World Out of Balance* (New York: Penguin, 1994), 398.

145   **14 of the first 408 cases:** Garrett, *The Coming Plague*, 397.

145   **Articles in the popular press:** Candice Belanoff and Philip Alcabes, "Toxic Shock Syndrome in the Popular Press, 1980–1990," abstract no. 28778, presented at the annual meeting of the American Public Health Association, Atlanta, October 23, 2001.

145   **American Legion convention:** CDC, reprinted from the January 18, 1977, special issue of *Morbidity and Mortality Weekly Report*, "Epidemiologic Notes and Reports Follow-up on Respiratory Illness—Philadelphia," *Morbidity and Mortality Weekly Report* 46, no. 3 (January 24, 1997): 50–56.

145   **isolated in early 1977:** J. E. McDade, C. C. Shepard, and D. W. Fraser, et al., "Legionnaires' Disease: Isolation of a Bacterium and Demonstra-

tion of Its Role in Other Respiratory Disease," *New England Journal of Medicine* 297 (1977): 1197.

146   **"A new human disease":** Garrett, *The Coming Plague*, 190.

146   **cases going back to 1947:** J. E. McDade, D. J. Brenner, and F. M. Bozeman, "Legionnaires' Disease Bacterium Isolated in 1947," *Annals of Internal Medicine* 90, no. 4 (April 1979): 659–661.

146   **as early as 1957:** Michael T. Osterholm, Tom D.Y. Chin, Donald O. Osborne, H. Bruce Dull, et al., "A 1957 Outbreak of Legionnaires' Disease Associated with a Meat Packing Plant," *American Journal of Epidemiology* 117 (1983): 60–67.

146   **stored water supply:** CDC, "Legionellosis: Legionnaire's Disease and Pontiac Fever," October 2005, at http://www.cdc.gov/legionella/patient _facts.htm (downloaded December 14, 2008).

147   **AIDS was recognized officially:** CDC, "Pneumocystis Pneumonia— Los Angeles," *Morbidity and Mortality Weekly Report* 30, no. 21 (June 5, 1981): 250–252.

147   **gay press in New York:** Larry Mass, "Cancer Hits the Gay Community," *New York Native*, July 12–28, 1981.

147   **"the umpteenth time":** Harold Ross, "Playing It Safe," *New York Native*, May 4–17, 1981.

148   **immune dysregulation:** Ann Giudici Fettner and William Check, *The Truth About AIDS*, revised ed. (New York: Holt, Rinehart and Winston, 1985), chaps. 1–2; Randy Shilts, *And the Band Played On* (New York: St. Martin's, 1987), part III.

148   **segued into research:** Michelle Cochrane, *When AIDS Began: San Francisco and the Making of an Epidemic* (New York: Routledge, 2004), 24. Information on investigators' state of mind was provided to me by a physician who was with the Epidemic Intelligence Service at the time.

148   **the Epidemic Intelligence Service officer in Los Angeles:** Giudici Fettner and Check, *The Truth About AIDS*, 15.

148   **the epidemiologist in the San Francisco health department:** Cochrane, *When AIDS Began*, 26.

148   **investigators felt their theories:** Shilts, *And the Band Played On*, 65–69 (1988 Penguin ed.). Shilts claims that CDC officials were concertedly putting the kibosh on the story in order to preclude news making by the gay movement.

149   **"for the most part unfounded":** Larry Mass, "The Epidemic Continues: Facing a New Case Every Day Researchers Are Still Bewildered," *New York Native*, March 29–April 11, 1982.

149   **first report on five cases:** CDC, "Pneumocystis Pneumonia," 250–252.

149 immune impairment: "'Gay' Pneumonia? Not Really, Says Researcher," *The Advocate*, July 23, 1981.

149 "risk factor": Larry Mass, "An Epidemic Q&A," *New York Native*, May 24–June 1, 1982.

149 By the time the new disease was named AIDS: The new name first appeared in the CDC publication *Morbidity and Mortality Weekly Reports* in September 1982. See "Current Trends: Update on Acquired Immune Deficiency Syndrome (AIDS)—United States," *Morbidity and Mortality Weekly Report* 31, no. 37 (September 24, 1982): 507–508, 513–514.

150 593 individuals: Ibid.

150 "sexual voracity": Susan Sontag, *Illness as Metaphor and AIDS and Its Metaphors* (New York: Anchor/Doubleday, 1990), 164.

150 homosexual "plague": Dennis Altman, *AIDS in the Mind of America* (Garden City: Anchor, 1986), 17–19; James Kinsella, *Covering the Plague: AIDS and the American Media* (New Brunswick: Rutgers, 1989), 54; "Homosexual Plague Strikes New Victims," *Newsweek*, August 23, 1982. Altman names several of the 1982 news articles; he gives August 9, 1982, as the date of the first article about "gay plague." Kinsella cites a syndicated article by United Press International writer Jan Ziegler that appeared in September 1982.

150 risk groups: CDC, "Update on Acquired Immune Deficiency Syndrome (AIDS)" (September 24, 1982).

151 "plague of medical jargon": Steven Harvey, *Village Voice*, December 21, 1982.

151 Larry Kramer charged: Larry Kramer, "1,112 and Counting," *New York Native*, March 14–27, 1982.

151 James Curran: James Curran, "Epidemiologic Aspects of the Current Outbreak of Kaposi's Sarcoma and Opportunistic Infections," *New England Journal of Medicine* 306, no. 4 (1982): 248–252. Curran's role in this article was made clear by Larry Mass in "The Epidemic Continues."

152 useful in the political debates: A discussion of the many understandings of "risk" in the context of the search for the causes of AIDS, and the political ramifications of the diversity of meanings of risk, is offered by Steven Epstein in *Impure Science: AIDS, Activism and the Politics of Knowledge* (Berkeley: University of California Press, 1996), 55–61.

153 "promiscuity": J. Sonnabend, "Promiscuity Is Bad for Your Health," *New York Native*, September 13–26, 1982.

153 another opinion piece: M. Callen and J. Berkowitz, "Two Men Declare War on Promiscuity," *New York Native*, November 8, 1982.

153   **recommended that gay men reduce:** American Association of Physicians for Human Rights, "Statement on AIDS and Healthful Gay Male Sexual Activity," *The Advocate*, April 28, 1983, 10.

153   **"AIDS crisis has given":** Nathan Fain, "Coping with a Crisis: AIDS and the Issues it Raises," *The Advocate*, February 17, 1983.

153   **far more effectively:** M. G. Hudgens, I. M. Longini Jr., S. Vanichseni, D. H. Hu, et al., "Subtype-Specific Transmission Probabilities for Human Immunodeficiency Virus Among Injecting Drug Users in Bangkok, Thailand," *American Journal of Epidemiology* 155 (2002): 159–168; R. A. Royce, A. Sena, W. Cates Jr., and M. S. Cohen, "Sexual Transmission of HIV," *New England Journal of Medicine* 336 (1997): 1072–1078.

153   **initial infection occurred:** Based on the timing of early cases of AIDS; limited data on the prevalence of HIV infection among New York City drug users entering treatment provided by Des Jarlais, et al., "HIV-1 Infection Among Intravenous Drug Users in Manhattan, New York City, from 1977 through 1987," JAMA 261, no. 7 (February 17, 1989): 1008–1012; and reports in the 1970s of unexplainable infections among drug users in and around New York City.

154   **practice of concurrent partnerships:** The consequences of concurrency are amply documented in Helen Epstein, *The Invisible Cure: Africa, the West, and the Fight Against AIDS* (New York: Farrar, Straus and Giroux, 2007).

154   **Dr. Otis Bowen:** Associated Press, "AIDS May Dwarf the Plague," *New York Times*, January 30, 1987.

155   **15,000 men visited the baths:** Gabriel Rotello, *Sexual Ecology: AIDS and the Destiny of Gay Men* (New York: Dutton, 1997), 62.

155   **men who had sex with more than 500 other men:** Ibid.

155   **multiple sexual exposures:** J. Sonnabend, "The Etiology of AIDS," *AIDS Research* 1, no. 1 (1983): 2–3.

155   **"but the victim of AIDS":** L. Mass, "Why the Baths Must Not Be Closed," quoted in Nathan Fain, "Coping with a Crisis: AIDS and the Issues It Raises."

155   **"not to have sex in the traditional sense of the word":** Randy Shilts, "A Possible 600 New AIDS Cases Expected in Area," *San Francisco Chronicle*, March 5, 1984.

155   **set a model for the nation:** Cited in Ronald Bayer, *Private Acts, Social Consequences: AIDS and the Politics of Public Health* (New Brunswick: Rutgers, 1989), 48.

155   **two gay bookstores:** The history of the ensuing controversy over bathhouse closure has been amply documented. See Rotello, *Sexual Ecology*,

chaps. 2 and 3; Bayer, *Private Acts, Social Consequences*, chap. 2; and Shilts, *And the Band Played On*, part I.

156   **closure would have no effect:** Bayer, *Private Acts, Social Consequences*, 42, 49–51.

156   **in the city's government:** Ibid., 52.

156   **"reap the whirlwind":** Cited in Shilts, *And the Band Played On*, 347.

156   **new epidemic was defined in terms of prudence:** Sontag, *Illness as Metaphor and AIDS and Its Metaphors*, 113, 144.

157   **a gay "holocaust":** Kramer, Larry, *Reports from the Holocaust: The Story of an AIDS Activist*, expanded edition (New York: St. Martin's, 1994).

157   **"transmitting death":** Pat Buchanan, syndicated op-ed column, May 24, 1983, cited in Shilts, *And the Band Played On*, 312.

157   **lack of "social capital":** D. R. Holtgrave and R. A. Crosby, "Social Capital, Poverty, and Income Inequality as Predictors of Gonorrhoea, Syphilis, Chlamydia and AIDS Case Rates in the United States," *Sexually Transmitted Infections* 79 (2003): 62–64; Holtgrave, Crosby, G. M. Wingood, R. J. DiClemente, and J. A. Gayle, "Social Capital as a Predictor of AIDS Cases, STD Rates and Adolescent Sexual Risk Behavior Prevalence: A State-Level Analysis, U.S.A., 1999," abstract no. ThOrD1493, presented at the International Conference on AIDS, July 7–12, 2002; and Robert D. Putnam, *Bowling Alone* (New York: Simon & Schuster, 2000).

158   **"logic behind temporary closure":** Cited in Bayer, *Private Acts, Social Consequences*, 56.

158   **"moderate restriction in civil liberties":** Gabriel Rotello, quoted in *Out* magazine, 1995, cited in John-Manuel Andriote, *Victory Deferred: How AIDS Changed Gay Life in America* (Chicago: University of Chicago Press, 1999), 161.

159   **"why not criminalize":** Letter by Stoddard, cited by Bayer, *Private Acts, Social Consequences*, 55.

159   **more research and treatment:** The history of the gay movement in relation to AIDS is nowhere better recounted than in Andriote's *Victory Deferred*.

160   **Officials modified the name to HIV/AIDS:** To my knowledge, the first public use of "HIV/AIDS" was by officials speaking at the 1988 International AIDS Conference in Stockholm; the new term appeared in three *New York Times* articles that summer, and it caught on from there.

161   **diagnosis by blood test:** CDC, "Update: Acquired Immunodeficiency Syndrome—United States," *Morbidity and Mortality Weekly Report* 36, no. 31 (August 14, 1987): 522–526.

161   **Needle- and syringe-exchange programs:** J. Normand, D. Vlahov, and L. E. Moses, eds., *Preventing HIV Transmission: The Role of Sterile Needles and Bleach* (Washington, DC: National Academy, 1995).

162   **omnibus spending legislation:** Kaiser Family Foundation, Kaiser Daily HIV/AIDS Report, February 5, 2008, compiled from *Washington Post*, *New York Times*, and other news sources, at http://www.kaisernetwork .org/daily_reports/rep_index.cfm?hint=1&DR_ID=50209 (downloaded December 14, 2008). Information on the omnibus spending bill of 2008, H.R. 2764, is available at the Library of Congress Web site for the 110th Congress, http://thomas.loc.gov/bss/d110query.html (downloaded January 13, 2009).

162   **gay men felt they had to:** Andriote, *Victory Deferred*, chap. 4.

163   **"woefully inadequate":** Ibid., 139–141.

163   **"frank, open discussions on AIDS":** Phillip M. Boffey, "Surgeon General Urges Frank Talk to Young on AIDS," *New York Times*, October, 23, 1986.

163   **"Don't die of ignorance":** U.K. Bureau of Hygiene & Tropical Diseases, *AIDS Newsletter* 2, no. 1 (January 15, 1987).

163   **continued to include:** The term "risk behavior" went into use circa 1990. See, for instance, J. A. Kelly, J. S. St. Lawrence, T. L. Brasfield, et al., "AIDS Risk Behavior Patterns Among Gay Men in Small Southern Cities," *American Journal of Public Health* 80, no. 4 (April 1990): 416–418; M. J. Rotheram-Borus, C. Koopman, C. Haignere, and M. Davies, "Reducing HIV Sexual Risk Behaviors Among Runaway Adolescents," *JAMA* 266, no. 9 (September 4, 1991): 1237–1241.

163   **Risky behavior was said to be the cause of AIDS:** For an early use of the term, see Gina Kolata, "Erotic Films in AIDS Study Cut Risky Behavior," *New York Times*, November 3, 1987.

163   **overheated discussion:** U.S. Substance Abuse and Mental Health Services Administration, *Alcohol, Drugs, and HIV/AIDS: A Consumer Guide*, DHHS publication SMA-06-4127 (2006), at http://kap.samhsa .gov/products/brochures/pdfs/HIVBroch(General).pdf (downloaded February 28, 2008).

164   **The archdiocese of New York:** A historical review of the condom wars in New York City's public schools is provided by Patricia Siplon in *AIDS and the Policy Struggle in the United States* (Washington, DC: Georgetown University Press, 2002), 76–80.

165   **The altar of safe sex:** In *Sexual Ecology*, Rotello recounts differing responses to the advice about condoms among various factions of gay activists in the mid-1980s and suggests that the condom campaign was part of an effort in which some activists participated, to "de-gay" AIDS.

166   **if everyone adopted the recommended behavior:** Several studies
among heterosexual populations showed that using condoms all the
time is very effective, whereas using them less than all the time allows
for high transmission rates. In a study of uninfected women who were
sex partners of HIV-positive men, HIV incidence rates were 1.1 percent per year among consistent users of condoms and 9.7 percent per
year among inconsistent or nonusers; in another study there were 10
infections among 104 initially uninfected partners of HIV-infected
heterosexuals who used condoms less than all the time, compared to
none among 100 couples who used condoms 100 percent of the time.
See A. Saracco, M. Musicco, A. Nicolosi, et al., "Man-to-Woman Sexual Transmission of HIV: Longitudinal Study of 343 Steady Partners of
Infected Men," *Journal of the Acquired Immune Deficiency Syndrome* 6
(1993): 497–502; and I. DeVincenzi and R. Ancelle-Park, "Heterosexual Transmission of HIV: Follow-up of a European Cohort of Couples,"
Proceedings of the Seventh International Conference on AIDS, Florence,
Italy, 1991, abstract MC3028. Transmission rates were high among
people who used condoms frequently but not all the time in a study by
I. De Vincenzi, "A Longitudinal Study of Human Immunodeficiency
Virus Transmission by Heterosexual Partners," *New England Journal of
Medicine* 331 (1994): 341–346; and another study by M. Guimarães,
et al., "HIV Infection Among Female Partners of Seropositive Men in
Brazil," *American Journal of Epidemiology* 142 (1995): 538–547.

166   **report of the death of a twenty-month-old child:** CDC, "Epidemio-
logic Notes and Reports: Possible Transfusion-Associated Acquired
Immune Deficiency Syndrome, AIDS-California," *Morbidity Mortality
Weekly Report* 31, no. 48 (December 10, 1982): 652–654.

166   **Scandals . . . contributed to the outcry:** The full history of controversy over the safety of the blood supply in the context of AIDS is provided in Eric Feldman and Ronald Bayer, eds., *Blood Feuds: AIDS,
Blood, and the Politics of Medical Disaster* (New York: Oxford, 1999). A
close analysis of the early debates over the safety of the U.S. blood supply appears in Bayer, *Private Acts, Social Consequences*, chap. 3.

166   **made its way through the courts:** J. Nundy, "Cambridge Don Charged
in AIDS Contamination Case," *Independent*, November 11, 1991;
Nundy, "Blood and Money," *Independent* magazine, November 23,
1991; S. Wavell, "Patients Pillory Doctor in HIV Blood Scandal," *Sunday Times* (London), June 13, 1992; A. Bell, "French AIDS Blood
Scandal Spreads, *Guardian*, July 25, 1992; and Bell and P. Webster,
"Blood Stains French Image of Justice," *Guardian*, October 24, 1992.

166   **nominally about the "ethics":** *Wadleigh v. Rhone-Poulenc*, originally filed in October 1993, was a class-action lawsuit on behalf of individuals with hemophilia infected with the AIDS virus by administration of blood products. Federal circuit court judge John Grady certified the plaintiffs as a class, but circuit court judge Richard Posner overturned on appeal, decertifying, and ultimately leading to an out-of-court settlement. In Siplon's account (*AIDS and the Policy Struggle in the United States*, 60–61), Judge Posner named several concerns, including the unlikelihood of plaintiff's victory since the defendant companies and foundation had won more than 90 percent of court cases against them.

167   **syringes were allowed:** Siplon, *AIDS and the Policy Struggle*, 80–86; Ernest Drucker, "Harm Reduction: A Public Health Strategy," *Current Issues in Public Health* 1 (1995): 64–70; E. Drucker, Peter Lurie, Alex Wodak, and Philip Alcabes, "Measuring Harm Reduction: The Effects of Needle and Syringe Exchange Programs and Methadone Maintenance on the Ecology of HIV," *AIDS* 12, supplement A (1998): S217–S230.

168   **Britain's Princess Anne:** Virginia Berridge, *AIDS in the UK: The Making of Policy, 1981–1994* (Oxford: Oxford, 1996), 163.

168   **those who are not innocent:** Sontag, *Illness as Metaphor and AIDS and Its Metaphors* (New York: Anchor/Doubleday, 1990), 99.

169   **Gaetan Dugas:** Shilts, *And the Band Played On*, 22–23, 38, 83–84. Shilts claims that he does not think that Dugas was the one person who brought the AIDS virus to America, but he is slippery about this belief. Compare pages 22 and 84 with page 439.

170   **race pervaded:** Andriote, *Victory Deferred*. Race is discussed repeatedly in Andriote's recounting of the AIDS story among American gays. Also see Cathy J. Cohen's insightful *Boundaries of Blackness: AIDS and the Breakdown of Black Politics* (Chicago: University of Chicago Press, 1999).

170   **assign a biological foundation:** Troy Duster, "The Molecular Reinscription of Race: Unanticipated Issues in Biotechnology and Forensic Science," *Patterns of Prejudice* 40, issues 4 and 5 (2006): 427–441.

171   **minority groups would not be served:** Andriote, *Victory Deferred*, 146–148.

171   **National Task Force for AIDS Prevention:** Ibid., 148.

171   **The DL phenomenon:** Benoit Denizet-Lewis, "Double Lives on the Down Low," *New York Times*, August 3, 2003; Sheryl Johnson, "The Lowdown on the 'Down Low,'" *AIDS Survival Project*, January/February 2004, at http://www.thebody.com/content/whatis/art32425.html (downloaded March 4, 2008).

171   **The myth of specialness:** CDC, "Questions and Answers: Men on the Down Low," April 12, 2006, updated October 19, 2006. Text is reproduced at http://www.thebody.com/index/whatis/down_low.html (downloaded December 14, 2008).

172   **open secrets:** David F. Greenberg, *The Construction of Homosexuality* (Chicago: University of Chicago Press, 1988), 316, 324–328, 330.

172   **homosexual cruising grounds:** Greenberg, *The Construction of Homosexuality*, 355.

172   **both single and married men:** George Chauncey, *Gay New York: Gender, Urban Culture, and the Making of the Gay Male World 1890–1940* (New York: Basic Books, 1994), quoted in Rotello, *Sexual Ecology*, chap. 2.

172   **stupid or injudicious:** JoAnn Wypijewski, "The Secret Sharer: Sex, Race, and Denial in an American Small Town," *Harper's*, July 1998, 35–56.

173   **sexual "depravity":** Christopher Farah, "AIDS: The Black Plague," review of *The Secret Plague: The Story of AIDS and Black America*, by Jacob Levenson. *Salon*, March 10, 2004, at http://dir.salon.com/story/ books/int/2004/03/10/levenson (downloaded March 11, 2008). Farah writes that the secret epidemic among black Americans is more than just AIDS; it is an epidemic of "human and sexual depravity."

173   **"monster":** The definitive account of the most infamous such incident is Thomas Shevory's *Notorious H.I.V.: The Media Spectacle of Nushawn Williams* (Minneapolis: University of Minnesota Press, 2004). See 16 for a compendium of epithets.

173   **"lethal lothario":** Wypijewski, "The Secret Sharer."

173   **"walking epidemic":** Donn Esmonde, "Existing Laws Aren't Enough for a Walking Epidemic," *Buffalo News*, October 29, 1997, cited in Shevory, *Notorious H.I.V.*, 16.

173   **"the bogeyman incarnate":** Rick Hampson, "AIDS Scare Rips Through Upstate N.Y.," *USA Today*, October 29, 1997, cited in Shevory, *Notorious H.I.V.*, 16.

173   **178 years in prison:** Associated Press, "Man Gets 178 Years for HIV Assaults," December 23, 2004, at http://www.spokesmanreview.com/ tools/story_pf.asp?ID=44574 (downloaded December 14, 2008).

173   **first-degree murder charges:** "HIV-Positive Man to Stand Trial on Murder Charges," CBC News, November 14, 2005, at http://www.amren .com/mtnews/archives/2005/11/hivpositive_man_to_stand_trial.php (downloaded December 14, 2008); "HIV Infected Man Who Lied to Sex Partners Sent to Prison for 56 Months," *Canadian Press*, January 20, 2007.

174   **"fine and courageous":** Ira Berkow, "Magic Johnson's Legacy," *New York Times*, November 8, 1991.

174   **"a victim, not a hero":** Dave Anderson, "Sorry, but Magic Isn't a Hero," *New York Times*, November 14, 1991.

174   **widespread sympathy for Johnson's "plight":** "Sympathy Overwhelming for Johnson's Plight," *USA Today*, November 8, 1991.

174   **certain that he contracted:** See, for instance, Doug Smith, "Magic Tells His Side, Denies Bisexual Rumors," *USA Today*, November 13, 1991.

174   **"most people are coming up negative":** "Johnson Searching for Source," *Financial Post* (Toronto), December 12, 1991.

175   **Apollonian-Dionysian dance:** Friedrich Nietzsche, *The Birth of Tragedy* (1872), trans. Francis Golffing (Garden City: Doubleday, 1956).

176   **doubling every fifteen to twenty months:** New York City Department of Health, "Surveillance Update, Including Persons Living with AIDS in New York City," semiannual report, 2002. See summary, "AIDS Diagnoses and Persons Living with HIV/AIDS by Year," at http://www.nyc.gov/html/doh/downloads/pdf/ah/surveillance2006_trend_tables.pdf (downloaded January 20, 2008).

176   **commissioner explained that the case:** New York City Department of Health and Mental Hygiene, "New York City Resident Diagnosed with Rare Strain of Multi-Drug Resistant HIV That Rapidly Progresses to AIDS," press release, February 11, 2005, at http://www.nyc.gov/html/doh/html/pr/pr016-05.shtml (downloaded December 14, 2008).

176   **"whether this [occurrence] . . . drug-resistant strains":** Lawrence Altman, "A Public Health Quandary: When Should the Public Be Told?" *New York Times*, February 15, 2005.

177   **"just a sin in our society":** Richard Pérez-Peña and Marc Santora, "AIDS Report Brings Alarm, Not Surprise," *New York Times*, February 13, 2005.

177   **two such cases had been reported in Vancouver:** C. Skelton, "New HIV 'Superbug' Emerges in Vancouver," *Vancouver Sun*, August, 9, 2001.

177   **Both of the earlier cases:** D. Brown, "Scope of Unusual HIV Strain Is Unknown, Experts Say," *Washington Post*, February 13, 2005.

177   **decried the announcement:** Frank Jordans, "Swiss Change Safe Sex Message on HIV," Associated Press online, January 31, 2008, at http://www.foxnews.com/wires/2008Jan31/0,4670,SwitzerlandAIDS,00.html (downloaded December 14, 2008).

178   **more than 2 million:** Joint United Nations Programme on HIV/AIDS and World Health Organization, "AIDS Epidemic Update 2007," December 2007, at http://data.unaids.org/pub/EPISlides/2007/2007_epiupdate_en.pdf (downloaded January 21, 2008).

178   **cumulatively, between 67 million and 80 million:** Joint United Nations
      Programme on HIV/AIDS, "AIDS in Africa: Three Scenarios to 2025,"
      December 2006, at http://data.unaids.org/Publications/IRC-pub07/jc1058
      -aidsinafrica_en.pdf (downloaded January 21, 2008).

178   **500 million cases each year, more than 1 million annual deaths:**
      World Health Organization, "Malaria Fact Sheet," May 2007, at http://
      www.who.int/mediacentre/factsheets/fs094/en/index.html (downloaded
      December 14, 2008).

178   **tuberculosis (8.8 million new cases, 1.6 million deaths):** World Health
      Organization, "Tuberculosis Fact Sheet," March 2007, at http://www
      .who.int/mediacentre/factsheets/fs104/en/index.html (downloaded De-
      cember 14, 2008).

178   **Susan Sontag wondered:** Sontag, *Illness as Metaphor and AIDS and Its
      Metaphors*, 181.

CHAPTER 7: MANAGING THE IMAGINED EPIDEMIC

181   **Our concern with history:** W. G. Sebald, *Austerlitz*, trans. Anthea
      Bell (New York: Modern Library, 2001), 72.

181   **Fatality rates in Ebola outbreaks:** In outbreaks going back to the mid-
      1970s there have been more than 1,500 Ebola virus deaths. In the first
      large Ebola hemorrhagic fever outbreak, in 1976 in Yambuku, Zaire, 88
      percent of the 318 cases died; 50–65 percent died in smaller outbreaks in
      Sudan in 1976 and 1979. From 1994 through 1997, outbreaks in Gabon
      killed 55–75 percent of those who fell ill, and another large Zairean out-
      break (315 cases) again saw fatality rates of more than 80 percent. In a
      recent outbreak in the Democratic Republic of Congo in the fall of
      2007, there were 264 confirmed cases, 71 percent of them fatal; another
      in Uganda in the winter of 2008 produced 149 cases and continued
      through February 2008. On the Sudan outbreaks, see World Health Or-
      ganization, "Ebola Haemorrhagic Fever in Zaire, 1976," *Bulletin of the
      World Health Organization* 56, no. 2 (1978): 271–293; World Health Or-
      ganization, "Ebola Haemorrhagic Fever in Sudan, 1976," *Bulletin of the
      World Health Organization* 56, no. 2 (1978): 247–270; and R. C. Baron,
      J. B. McCormick, and O. A. Zubeir, "Ebola Virus Disease in Southern
      Sudan: Hospital Dissemination and Intrafamilial Spread," *Bulletin of the
      World Health Organization* 61, no. 6 (1983): 997–1003. On the Gabon
      outbreak, see A. J. Georges, E. M. Leroy, A. A. Renaud, et al., "Ebola
      Hemorrhagic Fever Outbreaks in Gabon, 1994–1997: Epidemiologic
      and Health Control Issues," *Journal of Infectious Diseases* 179 (1999):
      S65–S75. On the 1995 Congo outbreak, see A. S. Khan, F. K. Tshioko,

D. L. Heymann, et al., "The Reemergence of Ebola Hemorrhagic Fever, Democratic Republic of the Congo, 1995," *Journal of Infectious Diseases* 179 (1999): S76–S86. On the Uganda outbreak, see World Health Organization, "Ebola Outbreak Contained in Uganda" (February 22, 2008), at http://www.who.int/features/2008/ebola_outbreak/en/ (downloaded January 14, 2009).

182   **few if any human carriers:** The CDC claims there is no carrier state for Ebola but also reports that an individual in Liberia was found to have Ebola antibodies, indicating prior infection, without having been ill. See CDC, Special Pathogens Branch, *Ebola Hemorrhagic Fever Information Packet* 2002, 1, at http://www.cdc.gov/ncidod/dvrd/spb/mnpages/dispages/Fact_Sheets/Ebola_Fact_Booklet.pdf (downloaded March 4, 2008).

182   *Addressing Emerging Infectious Disease Threats:* The executive summary was published in CDC's *Morbidity and Mortality Weekly Report* 43, RR-5 (1994): 1–18.

183   **reports from the 1920s:** S. Adolphus Knopf, "Tuberculosis in Young Women," JAMA 90 (1928): 532–535.

183   **increased thirtyfold:** Anthony S. Fauci, Nancy A. Touchette, Gregory K. Folkers, "Emerging Infectious Diseases: A 10-Year Perspective from the National Institute of Allergy and Infectious Diseases," *Emerging Infectious Diseases* 11, no. 4 (2005): 519–525.

183   **proposed 2009 federal budget will cut that amount:** Infectious Disease Society of America, "President's FY 2009 Budget Will Leave Many Infectious Diseases Programs in Shock," press release, February 7, 2008, at http://www.idsociety.org/Content.aspx?id=9772 (downloaded December 15, 2008).

184   **presumption, articulated in books and editorials:** Ken W. Alibek and Stephen Handelman, *Biohazard: The Chilling True Story of the Largest Covert Biological Weapons Program in the World* (New York: Dell, 2000); Judith Miller, Stephen Engelberg, and William Broad, *Germs: Biological Weapons and America's Secret War* (New York: Simon & Schuster, 2001); Walter Laqueur, *The New Terrorism: Fanaticism and the Arms of Mass Destruction* (New York: Oxford University Press, 1999); Michael Osterholm and John Schwartz, *Living Terrors: What America Needs to Know to Survive the Coming Bioterrorist Catastrophe* (New York: Delacorte, 2000); Jessica Stern, *The Ultimate Terrorists* (Cambridge, MA: Harvard University Press, 1999).

184   **September 11 Commission:** National Commission on Terrorist Attacks Upon the United States, *9/11 Report: The Complete Investigation: The National Commission on Terrorist Attacks Upon the United States* (New York: St. Martin's, 2004).

184   **BioShield allocated:** Project Bioshield: Progress in the War on Terror, White House Web site, July 2004, at http://www.whitehouse.gov/infocus/ bioshield/bioshield2.html (downloaded December 16, 2008).

184   **allocated $1.5 billion in 2003–2004:** Ibid.

185   **"The age of bioterror is now":** Editorial, "Not Science Fiction," *Washington Post*, January 27, 2005.

185   **Atlantic Storm:** University of Pittsburgh Medical Center, Center for Biosecurity, Atlantic Storm documents, at http://www.atlantic-storm.org/ (downloaded June 9, 2008).

185   **Unit 731:** Daniel Barenblatt, *A Plague Upon Humanity: The Secret Genocide of Axis Japan's Germ Warfare Operation* (New York: HarperCollins, 2004).

185   **religious cult:** Miller, Engelberg, and Broad, *Germs*, 18–33.

185   **mortality in purposely created outbreaks:** Philip Alcabes, "The Bioterrorism Scare," *American Scholar* (Spring 2004); Miller, Engelberg, and Broad, *Germs*, chap. 1.

188   **inexplicable trick:** René Dubos, *Mirage of Health* (Garden City: Anchor, 1959), 31. A half-century ago the biologist and humanist René Dubos was wary of officials claiming to have made an impact when nature was changing. "When the tide is receding from the beach it is easy to have the illusion that one can empty the ocean by removing water with a pail," he wrote.

189   **Americans:** H. Mokdad, E. S. Ford, B. A. Bowman, et al., "Prevalence of Obesity, Diabetes, and Obesity-Related Health Risk Factors, 2001," *JAMA* 289, no. 1 (2003): 76–79.

189   **Europeans:** "Reducing Risks, Promoting Healthy Life," World Health Organization (WHO), 2002 annual report, at http://www.who.int/whr/ 2002/en/ (downloaded December 16, 2008); European Opinion Research Group, "Special Eurobarometer: Physical Activity," Brussels, Commission of the European Communities, 2003, cited in WHO European Action Plan for Food and Nutrition Policy 2007–2012, at http:// www.euro.who.int/obesity (downloaded December 16, 2008).

189   **developing countries:** D. Yach, D. Stuckler, and K. D. Brownell, "Epidemiologic and Economic Consequences of the Global Epidemics of Obesity and Diabetes," *Nature Medicine* (2006): 12, 62–66.

189   **"greatest public health challenges":** World Health Organization, Obesity in Europe Web page, May 2008, at http://www.euro.who.int/obesity (downloaded December 16, 2008).

189   **"epidemic proportions":** "The Surgeon General's Call to Action to Prevent and Decrease Overweight and Obesity," U.S. Department of Health and Human Services, Public Health Service, Office of the Sur-

geon General, 2001, at http://www.surgeongeneral.gov/topics/obesity/ (downloaded December 16, 2008).

190   **90 percent of Americans:** K. M. Flegal, B. I. Graubard, D. F. Williamson, and M. H. Gail, "Excess Deaths Associated with Underweight, Overweight, and Obesity," *JAMA* 293, no. 15 (2005): 1861–1867.

190   **34 percent of American adults:** C. L. Ogden, M. D. Carroll, M. A. McDowell, and K. M. Flegal, "Obesity Among Adults in the United States—No Change Since 2003–2004," National Center for Health Statistics data brief no. 1, 2007.

190   **up from 21 percent:** H. Mokdad, E. S. Ford, B. A. Bowman, et al., "Prevalence of Obesity, Diabetes, and Obesity-Related Health Risk Factors, 2001," *JAMA* 289, no. 1 (2003): 76–79.

190   **between 6 and 27 percent of European adults:** F. Branca, H. Nikogosian, and T. Lobstein, eds., "The Challenge of Obesity in the WHO European Region and the Strategies for Response" (WHO Regional Office for Europe, 2007), 20.

191   **Bad things will happen:** CDC, "Overweight and Obesity, Health Consequences," May 2007, at http://www.cdc.gov/nccdphp/dnpa/obesity/consequences.htm (downloaded December 16, 2008); World Health Organization, "What Are the Health Consequences of Being Overweight?" November 2006, at http://www.who.int/features/qa/49/en/index.html (downloaded December 16, 2008).

191   **metabolic syndrome:** E. S. Ford, W. H. Giles, and W. H. Dietz, "Prevalence of the Metabolic Syndrome Among US Adults: Findings From the Third National Health and Nutrition Examination Survey," *JAMA* 287 (2002): 356–359; R. Weiss, J. Dziura, T. S. Burgert, W. V. Tamborlane, et al., "Obesity and the Metabolic Syndrome in Children and Adolescents," *Obstetrical & Gynecological Survey* 59, no. 12 (2004): 822–824.

191   **"obesity-diabetes epidemic":** Editorial, "Childhood Obesity and a Diabetes Epidemic," *New England Journal of Medicine* 346 (2002): 854–855; F. Ashe-Goins, J. Fradkin, J. Miall, and M. D. Owens, "The Obesity and Diabetes Epidemic: The State of the Science and the Challenge to Public Health," Medscape Webcast, January 27, 2004, at http://www.medscape.com/viewprogram/2903 (viewed June 16, 2008); F. R. Kaufman, *Diabesity: The Obesity-Diabetes Epidemic That Threatens America—and What We Must Do to Stop It* (New York: Random House, 2005); S. Smyth and A. Heron, "Diabetes and Obesity: The Twin Epidemics," *Nature Medicine* 12 (2006): 75–80; D. Yach, D. Stuckler, and K. D. Brownell, "Epidemiologic and Economic Consequences of the Global Epidemics of Obesity and Diabetes," *Nature Medicine* 12 (2006): 62–66.

191   **do not show any clear cause-and-effect relation:** P. Campos, A. Saguy, P. Ernsberger, E. Oliver, and G. Gaesser, "The Epidemiology of Overweight and Obesity: Public Health Crisis or Moral Panic?" *International Journal of Epidemiology* 35 (2006): 55–60.

191   **112,000 American deaths:** K. Flegal, B. I. Graubard, D. F. Williamson, M. H. Gail, "Excess Deaths Associated Underweight, Overweight, and Obesity," *JAMA* 293, no. 15 (2005): 1861–1867.

191   **incomplete management of diabetes and/or hypertension:** K. Slynkova, D. M. Mannino, G. S. Martin, R. S. Morehead, and D. E. Doherty, "The Role of Body Mass Index and Diabetes in the Development of Acute Organ Failure and Subsequent Mortality in an Observational Cohort," *Critical Care* 10, R137 (2006): 1–9; E. H. Livingston and C. Y. Ko, "Effects of Obesity and Hypertension on Obesity-Related Mortality," *Surgery* 137, no. 1 (2005): 16–25.

192   **linked to cardiovascular problems:** P. Campos, et al., "The Epidemiology of Overweight and Obesity," 55–60.

192   **The effect of smoking:** Paul Campos, *The Obesity Myth: Why America's Obsession with Weight Is Hazardous to Your Health* (New York: Penguin, 2004), 30. Campos points out that thinner people might be more likely to die from smoking-related problems but might also be encouraged to smoke by a socially influenced desire to be thin, so it might be safer to stay heavy if getting thin means taking up smoking. Also, some conditions that smoking seems to promote, like cardiovascular disease, seem to be less dangerous among older adults with high body mass.

192   **even lower than people of "normal" weight:** The studies using the most sound methods found that mortality is lowest among people whose body-mass index falls in the 25–30 range. The highest death rates occur among people with very low BMI, below 18.5 or 19. See K. Flegal, et al., "Excess Deaths"; R. A. Durazu-Arvizu, D. L. McGee, R. S. Cooper, Y. Liao, and A. Luke, "Mortality and Optimal Body Mass Index in a Sample of the U.S. Population," *American Journal of Epidemiology* 147 (1998): 739–749; R. P. Troiano, E. A. Frongillo Jr, J. Sobal, and D. A. Levitsky, "The Relationship Between Body Weight and Mortality: A Quantitative Analysis of Combined Information from Existing Studies," *International Journal of Obesity* 20 (1996): 63–75.

193   **"husky" car seats:** "Obesity Threatens a Generation: Facts You Should Know," *Washington Post*, May 17, 2008.

193   **metabolic syndrome:** S. M. Grundy, H. B. Brewer, J. I. Cleeman, S. C. Smith Jr., and C. Lenfant, "Definition of Metabolic Syndrome: Report of the National Heart, Lung, and Blood Institute/American Heart Association Conference on Scientific Issues Related to Definition," *Cir-*

culation 109 (2004): 433–438; E. S. Ford, W. H. Giles, and W. H. Dietz, "Prevalence of the Metabolic Syndrome Among US Adults: Findings from the Third National Health and Nutrition Examination Survey," *JAMA* 287 (2002): 356–359; and M. Trevisan, J. Liu, F. B. Bahsas, and A. Menotti, "Syndrome X and Mortality: A Population-Based Study," *American Journal of Epidemiology* 148 (1998): 958–966.

194   **low self-esteem, poor school performance:** W. H. Dietz, "Health Consequences of Obesity in Youth: Childhood Predictors of Adult Disease," *Pediatrics* 101 (1998): 518–525.

194   **early death:** The first major paper to allege that high body mass conferred a mortality risk was J. E. Manson, W. C. Willett, M. J. Stampfer, G. A. Colditz, et al., "Body Weight and Mortality Among Women," *New England Journal of Medicine* 333, no. 11 (1995): 677–685. Also A. Must, J. Spadano, E. H. Coakley, A. E. Field, et al., "The Disease Burden Associated with Overweight and Obesity," *JAMA* 282 (1999): 1523–1529; D. B. Allison, K. R. Fontaine, J. E. Manson, J. Stevens, and T. B. Vanitallie, "Annual Deaths Attributable to Obesity in the United States," *JAMA* 282 (1999): 1530–1538; A. H. Mokdad, J. S. Marks, D. F. Stroup, and J. L. Gerberding, "Actual Causes of Death in the United States, 2000," *JAMA* 291 (2002): 1238–1245, correction published in *JAMA* 293 (2005): 298. The single paper with carefully refined methods for statistical estimation of the connection between high BMI and mortality was K. M. Flegal, B. I. Graubard, D. F. Williamson, and M. H. Gail, "Excess Deaths Associated with Underweight, Overweight, and Obesity," *JAMA* 293, no. 15 (2005): 1861–1867.

194   **an "outbreak" of obesity in West Virginia:** Gina Kolata, "C.D.C. Investigates Outbreak of Obesity," *New York Times*, June 3, 2005.

195   **"spread through social networks":** N. A. Christakis and J. H. Fowler, "The Spread of Obesity in a Large Social Network over 32 Years," *New England Journal of Medicine* 357, no. 4 (2007): 370–379.

195   **"affects all segments of society":** Greg Critser, *Fat Land: How Americans Became the Fattest People in the World* (New York: Houghton Mifflin, 2003); Anita Manning, "It Takes a Society to Treat Kids' Diabetes, Expert Says," *USA Today*, May 17, 2006.

195   **more common among the poor:** P. B. Goldblatt, M. E. Moore, and A. J. Stunkard, "Social Factors in Obesity," *JAMA* 192 (1965): 1039–1044; J. Sobal and A. J. Stunkard, "Socioeconomic Status and Obesity: A Review of the Literature," *Psychological Bulletin* 105 (1989): 260–275; and B. M. Popkin and P. Gordon-Larsen, "The Nutrition Transition: Worldwide Obesity Dynamics and Their Determinants," *International Journal of Obesity* 28 (2004): S2–S9.

195   **plumpness signaled wealth:** Gina Kolata, *Rethinking Thin: The New Science of Weight Loss—and the Myths and Realities of Dieting* (New York: Farrar, Straus and Giroux, 2008), 66–67. Kolata notes that Oprah Winfrey sets a prominent example for spending money to get thin.

195   **21 percent of adults who had finished college:** A. H. Mokdad, E. S. Ford, B. A. Bowman, W. H. Dietz, et al., "Prevalence of Obesity, Diabetes, and Obesity-Related Health Risk Factors," *JAMA* 289 (2003): 79.

195   **disparity was even greater:** C. L. Ogden, M. D. Carroll, M. A. McDowell, and K. M. Flegal, "Obesity Among Adults in the United States— No Statistically Significant Change Since 2003–2004," data brief no. 1, National Center for Health Statistics, CDC, November 2007.

196   **browbeaten into surgery:** Kolata, *Rethinking Thin*, 67–70.

196   **recommend diet and exercise:** Ibid., chaps. 1, 2, and 8.

196   **"negligence, disorder, and want of charity":** For the Privy Council's order of 1543 and the temperament of the plague time, see Paul Murray Slack, *The Impact of Plague in Tudor and Stuart England* (London: Routledge & Kegan Paul, 1985), 203.

196   **national programs:** Susan Levine and Lori Aratani, "Inertia at the Top: Belated, Patchy Response Further Hamstrung by Inadequate Federal Attention, Experts Say," *Washington Post*, May 19, 2008.

196   **"Social-Ecological Model":** CDC, "Overweight and Obesity: Social-Ecological Model," at http://www.cdc.gov/nccdphp/dnpa/obesity/state _programs/se_model.htm, May 22, 2007, (downloaded December 16, 2008).

196   **$75 million program of federal grants:** Levine and Aratani, "Inertia at the Top."

197   **no study on the topic:** A. J. Stunkard, "Beginners Mind: Trying to Learn Something About Obesity," *Annals of Behavioral Medicine* 13 (1991): 22, cited in Kolata, *Rethinking Thin*, 92.

197   **financial profitability or the costs of a food culture:** Institute of Medicine, "Progress in Preventing Childhood Obesity: How Do We Measure Up?" September 13, 2006, at http://www.iom.edu/CMS/3788/ 25044/36980.aspx (downloaded December 16, 2008).

198   **the right amount of exercise:** Kolata, *Rethinking Thin*, 190–191.

198   **inability to control one's appetite:** But people are paying attention to the economic structures, like food advertising and the layout of urban and suburban environments. And increasingly they make their case by invoking obesity to justify their call for reform. See, for instance, Michael Pollan, *In Defense of Food: An Eater's Manifesto* (New York: Penguin, 2008); Eric Schlosser, *Fast Food Nation: The Dark Side of the All-American Meal* (New York: Houghton Mifflin, 2001); Brendan

Gleeson and Neil Sipe, *Creating Child Friendly Cities* (London: Taylor & Francis, 2006); K. Booth, M. Pinkston, and W. Poston, "Obesity and the Built Environment," *Journal of the American Dietetic Association* 105, no. 5 (2003): 110–117; S. Cummins and S. Macintyre, "Food Environments and Obesity—Neighbourhood or Nation?" *International Journal of Epidemiology* 35, no. 1 (2006): 100–104; R. Ewing, T. Schmid, R. Killingsworth, A. Zlot, S. Raudenbush, "Relationship Between Urban Sprawl and Physical Activity, Obesity, and Morbidity," in J. M. Marzluff, E. Shulenberger, W. Endlicher, M. Alberti, et al., eds., *Urban Ecology: An International Perspective on the Interaction Between Humans and Nature* (New York: Springer US, 2008).

198   **Childhood obesity is an American national catastrophe:** Quotations in this paragraph reported by Susan Levine and Rob Stein, "Obesity Threatens a Generation," *Washington Post*, May 17, 2008.

199   **"biggest problem facing children today":** American Public Health Association (APHA), "Obesity and Overweight Children [*sic*]: The Hidden Epidemic," 2008, at http://www.apha.org/programs/resources/obesity/defaulttest.htm (downloaded December 16, 2008).

199   **deep roots:** APHA, "Roots of the Childhood Obesity Epidemic," at http://www.apha.org/programs/resources/obesity/proresobesityroot.htm (downloaded December 16, 2008).

199   **the APHA asserts:** The findings in the APHA's "Hidden Epidemic" report are based on numerous published studies, but few include research data. The ones that do were focused on exactly the parents-at-fault questions suggested in the report's text. See, for instance, J. Sandberg and S. Hofferth, "Changes in Children's Time with Parents: United States, 1981–1997," *Demography* 38, no. 3 (2001): 423–436; I. Lissau and T. Sorensen, "Parental Neglect During Childhood and Increased Risk of Obesity in Young Adulthood," *Lancet* 343, no. 8893 (February 1994), 324–327; F. McLellan, "Marketing and Advertising: Harmful to Children's Health," *Lancet* 360, no. 9938 (September 2002): 100; D. Neumark-Sztainer, P. Hannan, M. Story, J. Croll, and C. Perry, "Family Meal Patterns: Associations with Sociodemographic Characteristics and Improved Dietary Intake Among Adolescents," *Journal of the American Dietetic Association* 103, no. 3 (March 2003): 317–322.

200   **5 percent:** U.S. National Center for Health Statistics, "Prevalence of Overweight Among Children and Adolescents: United States, 2003–2004," 2005, at http://www.cdc.gov/nchs/products/pubs/pubd/hestats/overweight/overwght_child_03.htm (downloaded December 16, 2007).

200   **increasing in Europe:** F. Branca, H. Nikogosian, and T. Lobstein, eds., "The Challenge of Obesity in the WHO European Region and the

Strategies for Response," World Health Organization Regional Office for Europe, Copenhagen, 2007, 20–26.

200   **twice the prevalence:** T. Lobstein and R. Jackson-Leach, "Child Overweight and Obesity in the USA: Prevalence Rates According to IOTF Definitions," *International Journal of Pediatric Obesity* 2, no. 1 (2007): 62–64.

201   **usual method for diagnosing "overweight" in a child:** C. L. Ogden, S. Z. Yanovski, M. D. Carroll, and K. M. Flegal, "Epidemiology of Obesity," *Gastroenterology* 132, no. 6 (2007): 2087–2102; S. E. Barlow and W. H. Dietz, "Obesity Evaluation and Treatment: Expert Committee Recommendations, Maternal and Child Health Bureau, Health Resources and Services Administration and the Department of Health and Human Services," *Pediatrics* 102 (1998): E29.

201   **upper 5 percent of the IQ distribution:** Malcolm Gladwell explains the fallacy in "None of the Above: What IQ Doesn't Tell You About Race," *New Yorker*, December 17, 2007; also see W. T. Dickens and J. R. Flynn, "Heritability Estimates Versus Large Environmental Effects: The IQ Paradox Resolved," *Psychological Review* 108, no. 2 (2001): 346–369.

202   **National Institute on Child Health and Human Development:** U.S. National Institute on Child Health and Human Development, Health Education Web page, September 2006, at http://www.nichd.nih.gov/health/education (downloaded December 16, 2008).

202   **and "Food-Safe Schools":** CDC, Adolescent Health Information Web page, July 2008, at http://www.cdc.gov/node.do/id/0900f3ec801e457a (downloaded December 16, 2008). The "Food-Safe Schools" program appears on a page posted in August 2008 at http://www.cdc.gov/healthy youth/foodsafety/actionguide.htm (downloaded December 16, 2008).

204   **one child out of every 160:** J. Bertrand, A. Mars, C. Boyle, C. Bove, et al., "Prevalence of Autism in a United States Population: The Brick Township, New Jersey, Investigation," *Pediatrics* 108 (2001): 1155–1161; S. Chakrabarti and E. Fombonne, "Pervasive Developmental Disorder in Preschool Children," *JAMA* 285 (2001): 3093–3099; and S. Chakrabarti and E. Fombonne, "Pervasive Developmental Disorders in Preschool Children: Confirmation of High Prevalence," *American Journal of Psychiatry* 162, no. 6 (2005): 1133–1141.

204   **historical documents:** Roy Richard Grinker, *Unstrange Minds: Remapping the World of Autism* (New York: Basic Books, 2007), 52–53.

204   **keep them out of asylums:** M. Neve and T. Turner, "History of Child and Adolescent Psychiatry," chap. 24, in M. Rutter and E. Taylor, eds., *Child and Adolescent Pscyhiatry*, 4th ed. (New York: Blackwell, 2002), 382.

204   coined in 1912 by a Swiss psychiatrist: The first use of "autistic" was by the German psychiatrist Eugen Blueler. See Grinker, *Unstrange Minds*, 44.

204   Autism and Asperger's syndrome: W. Kanner, "Autistic Disturbances of Affective Contact," *Nervous Child* 2 (1943): 217–250; H. Asperger, "Die 'Autistischen Psychopathen' im Kindesalter," *Archiv für Psychiatrie und Nervenkrankheiten* 117 (1944): 76–136 (English translation available in Uta Frith, *Autism and Asperger Syndrome* [Cambridge: Cambridge University Press, 1991]).

205   psychiatry as a preventive of social instability: Nikolas Rose, "Psychiatry as a Political Science: Advanced Liberalism and the Administration of Risk," *History of the Human Sciences* 9, no. 2 (1996): 1–23.

205   we bowl alone: Robert D. Putnam argues that American society has undergone a profound movement away from community: see *Bowling Alone: The Collapse and Revival of American Community* (New York: Simon & Schuster, 2000), chaps. 6 and 13.

206   cannot be compared: Grinker, *Unstrange Minds*, chaps. 5–7.

206   well-justified fear rather than troubling anxiety: Sigmund Freud, *Beyond the Pleasure Principle*, trans. James Strachey (New York: W. W. Norton, 1975). Freud distinguishes between anxiety, which is based on an expectation of or preparation for an undetermined or not-yet-realized future danger, and fear, which is a response to a directly observable or definite present danger.

206   increased awareness of autism: Grinker, *Unstrange Minds*, 146–172.

206   as recently as the 1980s: C. J. Newschaffer, L. A. Croen, J. Daniels, E. Giarelli, et al., "The Epidemiology of Autism Spectrum Disorders," *Annual Review of Public Health* 28 (2007): 235–258.

206   4.7 per 10,000: E. Fombonne, "Epidemiologic Surveys of Autism and Other Pervasive Developmental Disorders: An Update," *Journal of Autism and Developmental Disorders* 33, no. 4 (2003): 365–382.

206   more effective and available: L. Wing, "Autism Spectrum Disorders: No Evidence For or Against an Increase in Prevalence," *British Medical Journal (BMJ)* 312 (1996): 327–328; J. P. Baker, "Mercury, Vaccines, and Autism: One Controversy, Three Histories," *American Journal of Public Health* 98, no. 2 (2008): 244–253.

207   three-quarters of new ASD diagnoses: S. Chakrabarti and E. Fombonne, "Pervasive Developmental Disorders in Preschool Children: Confirmation of High Prevalence," *American Journal of Psychiatry* 162, no. 6 (2005): 1133–1141.

208   A 2005 essay: Robert F. Kennedy Jr., "Deadly Immunity," *Rolling Stone*, June 30, 2005, 57–66.

209   **Thimerosal was no longer used:** Baker, "Mercury, Vaccines, and Autism."

209   **"leaky gut" allows toxins:** A. J. Wakefield, S. H. Murch, A. Anthony, J. Linnell, et al., "Ileal-Lymphoid-Nodular Hyperplasia, Non-Specific Colitis, and Pervasive Developmental Disorder in Children," *Lancet* 351 (1998): 637–641.

210   **"mental hygiene" movement:** Rose, "Psychiatry as a Political Science."

211   **the Individuals with Disabilities Education Act (IDEA):** The role of IDEA in shaping the autism epidemic is explored by Grinker, *Unstrange Minds*, 150.

212   **the Department of Education reported:** Individuals with Disabilities Education Act Web site, data tables at https://www.ideadata.org/PartB TrendDataFiles.asp, Table B2B, September 2007 (downloaded December 16, 2008).

212   **misreads what is largely just a different way:** The argument that autism represents not a disorder but a broad swath of a much broader spectrum of ways of thinking and communicating is sharply made by Grinker in *Unstrange Minds*.

EPILOGUE: THE RISK-FREE LIFE

215   **To prolong life:** Saul Bellow, *Ravelstein* (New York: Viking, 2000), 54.

218   **when our children are sick:** In *Hystories: Hysterical Epidemics and Modern Media* (New York: Columbia University Press, 1997), Elaine Showalter advances the theory that suffering makes us more vulnerable to the story line of epidemic threat based on fantasies of abuse or failure.

221   **"colonizes a segment of a novel future":** Anthony Giddens advances the basic argument about modernity in *The Consequences of Modernity* (Palo Alto: Stanford University Press, 1990) and examines the anxiety of the double edge in *Modernity and Self-Identity* (Palo Alto: Stanford, 1991).

222   **application of *Bacillus thuringiensis*:** Andrew Spielman and Michael D'Antonio, *Mosquito: A Natural History of Our Most Persistent and Deadly Foe* (New York: Hyperion, 2001), 22.

223   **modern plague:** At a press conference held August 4, 2004, New York senator Charles Schumer quoted Anthony Placido, special agent in charge in the New York Field Division of the U.S. Drug Enforcement Administration, as saying, "Methamphetamine abuse is spreading like a plague across the country."

223 **"There is risk going on out there"**: Perry Halkitis is quoted by Sarah Kershaw, "Syphilis Cases on the Increase in the City," *New York Times*, August 12, 2007.

224 **related to HIV risk**: For instance, a small study of gay men in Los Angeles found that existing HIV infection was more common among groups with more compared to less self-reported methamphetamine use. See S. Shoptaw and C. J. Reback, "Associations Between Methamphetamine Use and HIV Among Men Who Have Sex with Men: A Model for Guiding Public Policy," *Journal of Urban Health* 83, no. 6 (November 2006): 1151–1157.

224 **worse than the garden-variety strains**: P. Doshi, "Trends in Recorded Influenza Mortality: United States, 1900–2004," *American Journal of Public Health* 98, no. 5 (2008): 939–945.

225 **complacency in combating the nonexistent bird flu epidemic**: Alastair Sharp, "U.S. Pledges Extra $320 Million for Bird Flu Fight," Reuters, October 25, 2008, at http://news.yahoo.com/s/nm/20081025/hl_nm/us_birdflu_egypt;_ylt=AuJlC6YjxRwhFB_zr0gbVuEQ.3QA (downloaded October 26, 2008).

226 **Nature's bloody teeth**: Alfred, Lord Tennyson wrote "Tho' nature, red in tooth and claw / With ravine, shrieked against his creed" in Canto 56, lines 15–16 of his poem "In Memoriam A.H.H.," published in 1849.

SELECTED BIBLIOGRAPHY

Alexander, John T. *Bubonic Plague in Early Modern Russia: Public Health and Urban Disaster*. New York: Oxford University Press, 2003.

Alibek, Ken W., and Stephen Handelman. *Biohazard: The Chilling True Story of the Largest Covert Biological Weapons Program in the World*. New York: Dell, 2000.

Altman, Dennis. *AIDS in the Mind of America*. Garden City: Anchor, 1986.

Aly, Götz, Peter Chroust, and Christian Pross. *Cleansing the Fatherland: Nazi Medicine and Racial Hygiene*. Baltimore: Johns Hopkins University Press, 1994.

Andriote, John-Manuel. *Victory Deferred: How AIDS Changed Gay Life in America*. Chicago: University of Chicago Press, 1999.

Baldwin, Peter. *Contagion and the State in Europe, 1830–1930*. Cambridge: Cambridge University Press, 1999.

Barenblatt, Daniel. *A Plague Upon Humanity: The Secret Genocide of Axis Japan's Germ Warfare Operation*. New York: HarperCollins, 2004.

Barry, John M. *The Great Influenza: The Epic Story of the Deadliest Plague in History*. New York: Viking, 2004.

Bayer, Ronald. *Private Acts, Social Consequences: AIDS and the Politics of Public Health*. New Brunswick: Rutgers University Press, 1989.

Bendictow, Ole J. *The Black Death, 1346–1353: The Complete History*. Rochester: Boydell Press, 2004.

Benenson, Abram S., ed. *Control of Communicable Diseases in Man*. 15th ed. Washington, DC: American Public Health Association, 1990.

Berridge, Virginia. *AIDS in the UK: The Making of Policy, 1981–1994*. Oxford: Oxford University Press, 1996.

Black, Edwin. *War Against the Weak: Eugenics and America's Campaign to Create a Master Race*. New York: Four Walls Eight Windows, 2003.

Blackburn, Simon. *Ruling Passions: A Theory of Practical Reasoning*. Oxford: Clarendon, 1998.

Boeckl, Christine M. *Images of Plague and Pestilence: Iconography and Iconology.* Kirksville, MO: Truman State University Press, 2000.

Boghurst, William. *Loimographia: An Account of the Great Plague of London in Year 1665.* Joseph Frank Payne, ed. London: Shaw, 1894.

Bottin, Francesco, Giovanni Santinello, Philip Weller, and C. W. T. Blackwell, eds. *Models of the History of Philosophy.* Boston: Kluwer Academic Publishers, 1993.

Bowen, John. *A Refutation of Some of the Charges Against the Poor.* London: John Hatchard, 1837.

Brandt, Allan. *No Magic Bullet: A Social History of Venereal Disease in the United States Since 1880.* New York: Oxford University Press, 1985.

Brookes, Tim, and Omar A. Khan. *Behind the Mask: How the World Survived SARS, the First Epidemic of the 21st Century.* Washington, DC: American Public Health Association, 2005.

Brossollet, Jacqueline, and Henri Mollaret. *Pourquoi la Peste? Le Rat, La Puce et Le Bubon.* Paris: Gallimard, 1994.

Bruinius, Harry. *Better for All the World: The Secret History of Forced Sterilization and America's Quest for Racial Purity.* New York: Knopf, 2006.

Campos, Paul. *The Obesity Myth: Why America's Obsession with Weight Is Hazardous to Your Health.* New York: Penguin, 2004.

Cavengo, Vincenzo. *Il Lazzaretto: Storia di un Quartiere di Milano.* Milan, Italy: Nuove Edizioni Duomo, 1989.

Chase, Marilyn. *The Barbary Plague: The Black Death in Victorian San Francisco.* New York: Random House, 2003.

Chin, James, ed. *Control of Communicable Diseases Manual.* 17th ed. Washington, DC: American Public Health Association, 1999.

Cochrane, Michelle. *When AIDS Began: San Francisco and the Making of an Epidemic.* New York: Routledge, 2004.

Cohen, Cathy J. *Boundaries of Blackness: AIDS and the Breakdown of Black Politics.* Chicago: University of Chicago Press, 1999.

Cohen, Jeremy. *The Friars and the Jews: The Evolution of Medieval Anti-Judaism.* Ithaca: Cornell University Press, 1982.

Critser, Greg. *Fat Land: How Americans Became the Fattest People in the World.* New York: Houghton Mifflin, 2003.

Davies, Norman. *Europe: A History.* New York: Oxford University Press, 1996.

Dickens, Charles. *Hard Times.* Boston: Colonial Press, 1868. First American ed., 1854.

Drexler, Madeline. *The Menace of Emerging Infections.* New York: Penguin, 2003.

Dubos, René. *Mirage of Health.* Garden City: Anchor, 1959.

Duffy, John. *The Sanitarians: A History of American Public Health*. Urbana: University of Illinois Press, 1990.

Emerson, Ralph Waldo. *The Portable Emerson*. New York: Viking Press, 1946.

Engels, Friedrich. *The Condition of the Working Class in England*. 1846. Reprint, New York: Oxford University Press, 1993.

Epstein, Helen. *The Invisible Cure: Africa, the West, and the Fight Against AIDS*. New York: Farrar, Straus and Giroux, 2007.

Epstein, Steven. *Impure Science: AIDS, Activism and the Politics of Knowledge*. Berkeley: University of California Press, 1996.

Evans, R. J. W., and Hartmut Pogge von Strandmann, eds. *The Revolutions in Europe, 1848–1849: From Reform to Reaction*. Oxford: Oxford University Press, 2000.

Feldman, Eric, and Ronald Bayer, eds. *Blood Feuds: AIDS, Blood, and the Politics of Medical Disaster*. New York: Oxford University Press, 1999.

Feldberg, Georgina. *Disease and Class: Tuberculosis and the Shaping of Modern North American Society*. New Brunswick: Rutgers University Press, 1995.

Fettner, Ann Giudici, and William Check. *The Truth About AIDS: Evolution of an Epidemic*. Revised ed. New York: Holt, Rinehart and Winston, 1985.

Feyerabend, Paul. *Against Method: Outline of an Anarchistic Theory of Knowledge*. Revised ed. San Francisco: Analytical Psychology Club, 1988.

Francis, Mark. *Herbert Spencer and the Invention of Modern Life*. Ithaca: Cornell University Press, 2007.

Freud, Sigmund. *Beyond the Pleasure Principle*. Trans. James Strachey. New York: Norton, 1975.

Fuller, Steve. *Kuhn vs. Popper: The Struggle for the Soul of Science*. New York: Columbia University Press, 2004.

Garrett, Laurie. *Betrayal of Trust: The Collapse of Global Public Health*. New York: Hyperion, 2000.

———. *The Coming Plague: Newly Emerging Diseases in a World Out of Balance*. New York: Penguin, 1995.

Gaskell, Elizabeth. *Mary Barton*. London: Oxford University Press, 1906.

Giddens, Anthony. *The Consequences of Modernity*. Palo Alto: Stanford University Press, 1990.

———. *Modernity and Self-Identity*. Palo Alto: Stanford University Press, 1991.

Ginzburg, Carlo. *Ecstasies: Deciphering the Witches' Sabbath*. Trans. Raymond Rosenthal. New York: Penguin, 1991.

Glass, James M. *"Life Unworthy of Life": Racial Phobia and Mass Murder in Hitler's Germany*. New York: Basic, 1997.

Gleeson, Brendan, and Neil Sipe. *Creating Child Friendly Cities*. London: Taylor & Francis, 2006.

Gottfried, Robert. *The Black Death: Natural and Human Disaster in Medieval Europe*. New York: Free Press, 1983.

Greenberg, David F. *The Construction of Homosexuality*. Chicago: University of Chicago Press, 1988.

Grinker, Roy Richard. *Unstrange Minds: Remapping the World of Autism*. New York: Basic, 2007.

Habermas, Jürgen. *The Structural Transformation of the Public Sphere*. Trans. Thomas Berger. Cambridge: MIT Press, 1998.

Hays, J. N. *The Burdens of Disease: Epidemics and Human Response in Western History*. New Brunswick: Rutgers University Press, 2000.

Herring, Francis. *Certaine Rules, Directions, or Advertisements for This Time of Pestilentiall Contagion*. London: William Jones, 1625. Reprint, New York: Da Capo, 1973.

Hopkins, Donald R. *The Greatest Killer: Smallpox in History*. Chicago: University of Chicago Press, 2002.

Horrox, Rosemary. *The Black Death*. Manchester: Manchester University Press, 1994.

Howard, Michael. *The Franco-Prussian War: The German Invasion of France, 1870–1871*. New York: Routledge, 2001.

Jastrow, J. *Wish and Wisdom*. New York: Appleton-Century, 1935.

Jewish Publication Society, trans. *Tanakh: The Holy Scriptures*. Philadelphia: JPS, 1985.

Johnson, Charles S. *Shadow of the Plantation*. Chicago: University of Chicago Press, 1934.

Johnson, Steven. *The Ghost Map: The Story of London's Most Terrifying Epidemic and How It Changed Science, Cities, and the Modern World*. New York: Penguin, 2007.

Jones, James. *Bad Blood: The Tuskegee Syphilis Experiment*. Expanded ed. New York: Free Press, 1993.

Kaufman, F. R. *Diabesity: The Obesity-Diabetes Epidemic That Threatens America—and What We Must Do to Stop It*. New York: Random House, 2005.

Kelly, John. *The Great Mortality: An Intimate History of the Black Death, the Most Devastating Plague of All Time*. New York: Harper, 2005.

Kershaw, Ian. *Hitler, 1936–1945: Nemesis*. New York: Norton, 2000.

Kinsella, James. *Covering the Plague: AIDS and the American Media*. New Brunswick: Rutgers University Press, 1989.

Klee, Ernst. *"Euthanasie" im NS-Staat: Die "Vernichtung Lebensunwerten Lebens."* Frankfurt: Fischer, 1985.

Kolata, Gina. *Rethinking Thin: The New Science of Weight Loss—and the Myths and Realities of Dieting*. New York: Farrar, Straus and Giroux, 2008.

Kraut, Alan. *Silent Travelers: Germs, Genes, and the "Immigrant Menace."* Baltimore: Johns Hopkins University Press, 1994.

Laqueur, Walter. *The New Terrorism: Fanaticism and the Arms of Mass Destruction.* New York: Oxford University Press, 1999.

Leavitt, Judith Walzer. *Typhoid Mary: Captive to the Public's Health.* Boston: Beacon Press, 1996.

Levy-Bruhl, Lucien. *Primitives and the Supernatural.* London: Allen and Unwin, 1936.

Lifton, Robert Jay. *The Nazi Doctors: Medical Killing and the Psychology of Genocide.* New York: Perseus, 1986.

Lloyd, G. E. R. *In the Grip of Disease: Studies in the Greek Imagination.* New York: Oxford University Press, 2003.

Luker, Kristin. *When Sex Goes to School: Warring Views on Sex—and Sex Education—Since the Sixties.* New York: Norton, 2006.

Lyons, Maryinez. *The Colonial Disease: A Social History of Sleeping Sickness in Northern Zaire, 1900–1940.* New York: Cambridge University Press, 1992.

MacMahon, B., and T. F. Pugh. *Epidemiology: Principles and Methods.* Boston: Little, Brown, 1970.

Markel, Howard. *Quarantine! East European Jewish Immigrants and the New York City Epidemics of 1892.* Baltimore: Johns Hopkins University Press, 1997.

———. *When Germs Travel: Six Major Epidemics That Invaded America Since 1900 and the Fears They Unleashed.* New York: Pantheon, 2004.

Marks, Geoffrey, and William K. Beatty. *Epidemic.* New York: Scribner, 1976.

Martin, A. Lynn. *Plague? Jesuit Accounts of Epidemic Disease in the 16th Century.* Kirksville, MO: Truman State University Press, 1996.

McNeill, William H. *Plagues and Peoples.* New York: Anchor/Doubleday, 1977.

Miller, Judith, Stephen Engelberg, and William Broad. *Germs: Biological Weapons and America's Secret War.* New York: Simon & Schuster, 2001.

Morse, Stephen L. *Emerging Viruses.* New York: Oxford University Press, 1996.

Nohl, Johannes. *The Black Death: A Chronicle of the Plague Compiled from Contemporary Sources.* London: Unwin, 1961.

Normand, J., D. Vlahov, and L. E. Moses, eds. *Preventing HIV Transmission: The Role of Sterile Needles and Bleach.* Washington, DC: National Academy Press, 1995.

O'Shea, Stephen. *The Perfect Heresy: The Revolutionary Life and Death of the Medieval Cathars.* New York: Walker and Co., 2001.

Osterholm, Michael, and John Schwartz. *Living Terrors: What America Needs to Know to Survive the Coming Bioterrorist Catastrophe.* New York: Delacorte, 2000.

Parets, Miquel. *A Journal of the Plague Year: The Diary of the Barcelona Tanner Miquel Parets, 1651.* Trans. James S. Amelang. New York: Oxford University Press, 1991.

Pepys, Samuel. *The Diary of Samuel Pepys.* Vol. 6, Robert Latham and William Matthews, eds. Berkeley: University of California Press, 1972.

Pernick, Martin S. *The Black Stork: Eugenics and the Death of "Defective" Babies in American Medicine and Motion Pictures Since 1915.* New York: Oxford University Press, 1999.

Pollan, Michael. *In Defense of Food: An Eater's Manifesto.* New York: Penguin, 2008.

Porter, Dorothy. *Health, Civilization and the State: A History of Public Health from Ancient to Modern Times.* New York: Routledge, 1999.

Porter, Roy. *Bodies Politic: Disease, Death and Doctors in Britain, 1650–1900.* Ithaca: Cornell University Press, 2001.

———. *Flesh in the Age of Reason: The Modern Foundations of Body and Soul.* New York: Norton, 2003.

Porter, Stephen. *The Great Plague.* Phoenix Mill, UK: Stroud, 1999.

Proctor, Robert. *Racial Hygiene: Medicine Under the Nazis.* Cambridge: Harvard University Press, 1988.

Putnam, Robert D. *Bowling Alone: America's Declining Social Capital.* New York: Simon & Schuster, 2000.

Rather, L. J., ed. *Collected Essays in Public Health and Epidemiology.* Vol. 1. Boston: Science History Publications, 1985.

Reverby, Susan M., ed. *Tuskegee's Truths: Rethinking the Tuskegee Syphilis Study.* Chapel Hill: University of North Carolina Press, 2000.

Rhodes, Richard. *Masters of Death: The SS-Einsatzgruppen and the Invention of the Holocaust.* New York: Knopf, 2002.

Rogers, Naomi. *Dirt and Disease: Polio Before FDR.* New Brunswick: Rutgers University Press, 1996.

Rosen, George. *A History of Public Health.* Expanded ed. Baltimore: Johns Hopkins University Press, 1993.

Rosenberg, Charles E. *The Cholera Years.* Chicago: University of Chicago Press, 1962.

Rotello, Gabriel. *Sexual Ecology: AIDS and the Destiny of Gay Men.* New York: Dutton, 1997.

Ruffié, Jacques, and Jean-Charles Sournia. *Les Épidémies dans l'Histoire de l'Homme.* Paris: Flammarion, 1984.

Scheja, Georg. *The Isenheim Altarpiece.* Trans. by Robert Erich Wolf. New York: Harry N. Abrams, 1969.

Scherman, Nosson, ed. *The Tanach, Stone Edition.* 2nd ed. New York: Schocken, 1998.

Schlosser, Eric. *Fast Food Nation: The Dark Side of the All-American Meal.* New York: Houghton Mifflin, 2001.

Schmölzer, Hilde. *Die Pest in Wien.* Berlin: Verlag der Nation, 1988.

Scott, Susan, and Christopher J. Duncan. *Biology of Plagues: Evidence from Historical Populations.* Cambridge: Cambridge University Press, 2001.

Shevory, Thomas. *Notorious H.I.V.: The Media Spectacle of Nushawn Williams.* Minneapolis: University of Minnesota Press, 2004.

Shilts, Randy. *And the Band Played On: Politics, People, and the AIDS Epidemic.* New York: Penguin, 1988.

Showalter, Elaine. *Hystories: Hysterical Epidemics and Modern Media.* New York: Columbia University Press, 1997.

Siplon, Patricia. *AIDS and the Policy Struggle in the United States.* Washington, DC: Georgetown University Press, 2002.

Slack, Paul. *The Impact of Plague in Tudor and Stuart England.* Boston: Routledge and Kegan Paul, 1985.

———, ed. *The Plague Reconsidered: A New Look at Its Origins and Effects in 16th and 17th Century England.* Matlock, UK: Social Population Studies, 1977.

Smith, Herbert A. *A Letter to the Labouring Classes in Their Own Behalf.* London: W. Tyler, 1837.

Sontag, Susan. *Illness as Metaphor and AIDS and Its Metaphors.* New York: Anchor/Doubleday, 1990.

Spielman, Andrew, and Michael D'Antonio. *Mosquito: A Natural History of Our Most Persistent and Deadly Foe.* New York: Hyperion, 2001.

Starr, Paul. *The Social Transformation of American Medicine.* New York: Basic, 1982.

Stern, Jessica. *The Ultimate Terrorists.* Cambridge: Harvard University Press, 1999.

Tomes, Nancy. *The Gospel of Germs: Men, Women, and the Microbe in American Life.* Cambridge: Harvard University Press, 1998.

Trachtenberg, Joshua. *The Devil and the Jews: The Medieval Conception of the Jew and Its Relation to Modern Antisemitism.* Philadelphia: Jewish Publication Society, 1983.

Tuchman, Barbara. *A Distant Mirror: The Calamitous 14th Century.* New York: Knopf, 1978.

Washington, Harriet. *Medical Apartheid: The Dark History of Medical Experimentation on Black Americans from Colonial Times to the Present.* New York: Doubleday, 2007.

Watts, Sheldon. *Epidemics and History: Disease, Power and Imperialism.* New Haven: Yale University Press, 1997.

Wheelis, Mark, Lajos Rozsa, and Malcolm Dando, eds. *Deadly Cultures: Biological Weapons Since 1945.* Cambridge: Harvard University Press, 2006.

Winslow, Charles-Edward Amory. *The Conquest of Epidemic Disease: A Chapter in the History of Ideas*. 1943. Reprint, Madison: University of Wisconsin Press, 1980.

Ziegler, Philip. *The Black Death*. New York: John Day Co., 1969.

Ziermann, Horst. *Matthias Grünewald*. New York: Prestel Verlag, 2001.

INDEX

Accident, epidemics as, 24
Accidental death, 2–3
Achenwall, Gottfried, 94–95
Act of Settlement and Removal, 64
Addressing Emerging Infectious Disease
    Threats (CDC report), 182
The Advancement of Learning
    (Bacon), 67
African Americans
    AIDS as race issue, 170–175
    cholera as a product of
      intemperance and dissolution, 74
    forced sterilization of, 130–131
    genetic determinism, 132–133
    social Darwinism and germ theory,
      101–102
    syphilis as race issue, 134–137
AIDS
    American debut, 147–152
    applying blame for spread of, 52
    as crisis of identity and lifestyle,
      157–160
    as emerging infection, 182
    as gay plague, 21–22
    as race issue, 101–102, 137, 170–175
    behavior and homosexuality, 89,
      175–177
    cause and effect, 160–161
    education and prevention programs,
      161–165, 165–168

    epidemic rhetoric, 3
    health officials' roles as risk
      identifiers, 187
    highlighting discomfort with
      modernity, 177–180
    homosexuals as modern lepers, 30
    infection rate, 178
    literary symbolism, 2
    penitence as outgrowth of, 37
    predictions about, 228
    sanitizing public portrayal of,
      168–169
    sexual deviance debate, 154–160
    transmission of, 153–154, 160–161
Air quality
    Airplane Man tuberculosis incident,
      54–56
    as actual cause of illness, 53
    cholera in industrial Britain, 63
    cholera transmission theory, 66
    Legionnaires' disease, 145–146
    stench/odor, 66, 69-70, 75
    See also Miasma theory
Airline travel
    Airplane Man, 54–56
    SARS outbreak, 83–85
American Association of Physicians for
    Human Rights, 153
American Museum of Natural History,
    111–112

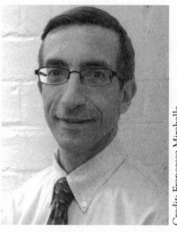

Credit: Francesca Mirabella

Philip Alcabes is an associate professor of Urban Public Health at Hunter College of the City University of New York and visiting clinical associate professor at the Yale School of Nursing. He has written op-eds for the *Washington Post* and contributed essays to *The American Scholar, Chronicle of Higher Education,* and *Virginia Quarterly Review.* He lives in the Bronx, New York.

PublicAffairs is a publishing house founded in 1997. It is a tribute to the standards, values, and flair of three persons who have served as mentors to countless reporters, writers, editors, and book people of all kinds, including me.

I. F. STONE, proprietor of *I. F. Stone's Weekly*, combined a commitment to the First Amendment with entrepreneurial zeal and reporting skill and became one of the great independent journalists in American history. At the age of eighty, Izzy published *The Trial of Socrates*, which was a national bestseller. He wrote the book after he taught himself ancient Greek.

BENJAMIN C. BRADLEE was for nearly thirty years the charismatic editorial leader of *The Washington Post*. It was Ben who gave the *Post* the range and courage to pursue such historic issues as Watergate. He supported his reporters with a tenacity that made them fearless and it is no accident that so many became authors of influential, best-selling books.

ROBERT L. BERNSTEIN, the chief executive of Random House for more than a quarter century, guided one of the nation's premier publishing houses. Bob was personally responsible for many books of political dissent and argument that challenged tyranny around the globe. He is also the founder and longtime chair of Human Rights Watch, one of the most respected human rights organizations in the world.

• • •

For fifty years, the banner of Public Affairs Press was carried by its owner Morris B. Schnapper, who published Gandhi, Nasser, Toynbee, Truman, and about 1,500 other authors. In 1983, Schnapper was described by *The Washington Post* as "a redoubtable gadfly." His legacy will endure in the books to come.

Peter Osnos, *Founder and Editor-at-Large*